Heterochronic Parabiosis

Anti-Aging Plasma Exchange

Fu-shih Pan,
M.D., Ph.D.

First Edition
Diplomate,
American Board Of
Plastic Surgery

Printed in Taiwan, Republic of China

For information address:

Elephant White Cultural Enterprise Ltd. Press,

8F.-2, No.1, Keji Rd., Dali Dist., Taichung City 41264, Taiwan (R.O.C.)

Distributed by Elephant White Cultural Enterprise Co., Ltd.

ISBN: 9786267018729

Suggested Price: NT$900

Contents

FOREWORD

I am pleased to have the opportunity to recommend this book which brings valuable pieces of information for the benefit of mankind.

I met Dr. Pan on a casual occasion through the introduction of a friend. Dr. Pan is an M.D. and Ph.D. in Chemistry, a reputable plastic surgeon, and a scientist. He has more than 40 years of experience in research and more than 30 years of experience in clinical medicine.

After I took charge of the Wan Hai Lines, I became a firm believer in "Health is Wealth" and have been receiving various anti-aging therapies*. When Dr. Pan explained the science behind heterochronic parabiosis, I immediately became interested and decided to receive the treatment. After only a few sessions, I felt my energy level had improved, the dark shadow of the skin around my toes resolved, and the pigmentation of my face had lightened up. My friends also noticed the changes in my appearance for which I have received many compliments. Since then I have become a great supporter of the plasma exchange program based on the principle of heterochronic parabiosis.

The most unique aspect of the book is that it is organized by a series of questions. Dr. Pan used these questions to guide the readers to explore the vast amount of information in the rapidly growing field of anti-aging medicine. If you read the book carefully, you will understand how scientists are approaching questions by asking one after another one of the questions, followed by carefully designed experiments and analysis of data collected, to find the answer.

The book starts from the basic concept of aging and explains the monumental work of Dr. Alexis Carrel who is the winner of the 1912 Nobel Prize in Physiology and Medicine. His works in connecting blood vessels of animals and organs of different ages using surgical techniques as well as further development of this method by Dr. Clive McCay set the scientific foundation of heterochronic parabiosis. These old-young pairing experiments revealed that the old animal becomes younger while the young animal becomes older in merely a few weeks. The results of these experiments are visible and are a fascinating phenomenon. This book continues by describing the scientific and clinical development of anti-aging technologies related to this old-young pair over the past 100 years.

This book also mentioned that during pregnancy, the mother and the baby shared the circulation via the umbilical cord and placenta, it is like heterochronic parabiosis except for the sizes of them are of great difference. Population statistics show that the chance of a mother who has her last children at age of 45 has a 50% higher chance of living to 80 years old as compared to women who have their last children 10 years younger at age of 35.

After I finished reading this book, I realized that heterochronic parabiosis is more than just an emerging anti-aging medical treatment, it is a science that is based on rigorous scientific principles as compared to medicine which is sometimes more of an art. Just like adding water to a cup of espresso will make it look and tastes lighter, is a science. Heterochronic parabiosis is a technology that makes the blood younger, when the blood becomes younger, the function of the cell will improve, and the aging phenomena are reversed.

If you are interested in the science of aging or anti-aging or want to delay the aging process of your body or improve aging-related diseases or are merely interested in the clinical application of the heterochronic parabiosis technology, I would recommend this book to you without any hesitation.

Understanding the problems associated with aging and exploring potential anti-aging science and technologies will not only resolve your curiosity and will benefit the health of yourself and your loved ones. I hope everyone who has had the chance to read this book enjoys a healthy life and longevity.

Dr. Ching-Chih Chen**
Group Chairman
Wan Hai Lines Ltd.

** Dr. Ching-Chih Chen is a B.S. in Physics and a Ph.D. in Economics from the Massachusetts Institute of Technology. He was a Professor in Economics at National Taiwan University and a consultant to the Ministry of Finance, Taiwan. He was the President of Wan Hai Lines Ltd. from 1969-1989 and Chairman from 1989-2008, during which he successfully built the company to become one of the largest players in the container shipping industry worldwide.

* Dr. Ching-Chih Chen has received the La Prairie Therapy annually from 1991 till 2000 for 9 consecutive years. He also had been to Morishita Clinic in Nagoya, Japan for placenta tissue therapy 3-4 times a year for 19 years. He began a modified version of intermittent fasting in 2019.

PREFACE

To live and look young forever has been the dream of mankind. Now, for the first time in history, the secret of aging and the method to reverse it has been revealed scientifically red

About 100 hundred years ago, scientists performed an experiment called heterochronic parabiosis to successfully reverse the aging phenomena of old animals in the laboratory. However, this method requires connecting the old animal to a young animal therefore is not feasible in any clinical setting.

Based on the effort of numerous scientists and physicians, the underlying mechanism of how heterochronic parabiosis reverses the aging phenomena has been decoded, several therapeutic options have also been described and attempted, and the results are very positive. The dream of extended healthspan and longevity as well as rejuvenation of degenerated functions of our aging body should become true very soon if not already so.

What is heterochronic parabiosis?

In short, it is the use of materials (e.g. blood, tissue extracts, or stem cells) obtained from young organisms to make the old organism young again.

Dr. Alexis Carrel performed a series of interesting experiments at my alma mater, the University of Chicago, during his tenure between 1904 and 1906. He was able to connect the vessels of an animal or its organ to another animal and kept it alive for weeks in time. By this technique, he was able to study the effect of aging and the mechanisms of other disease processes. This is the first time and the only experimental method to date where effects of aging reversal could be observed with naked eyes within days. Obviously, the technique could not be applied to humans. As a result, he started another series of experiments after relocating to Rockefeller University in maintaining the cells of the chicken heart in a culture dish using media obtained from chicken embryos for more than 30 years. Based on this, Dr. Carrel declared that the cell is immortal.

The findings of Carrel were largely forgotten due to the lack of clinical applications until the millennium when the baby boomers reached their age of retirement and became victims of chronic degenerative diseases. The social-economic impact was tremendous and attracted the attention of the government of all developed countries. As a result, academic institutions, pharmaceutical companies, and biotechnology start-ups or establishments all began to engage in the development of products and services to solve various problems associated with aging.

As a plastic surgeon with a practice focused on facelift procedures, I began to notice the loss of harmony in post-operative patients. This is resulting from the old skin relocated to a more youthful position. Although there were options like chemical peel, laser resurfacing, for the skin rejuvenation, these are not without significant side effects, e.g. hyperpigmentation, dermal thinning, etc... As a result, I became very interested in regenerative medical technologies that might rejuvenate the facial appearance in a natural way.

At that time, mesenchymal stem cells were isolated in the lipoaspirate of liposuction procedure. I went ahead to take a course in stem cell culture and eventually set up a company for isolation and culture stem cells obtained from the fat in Taipei, Taiwan and Penang, Malaysia. This also opened the opportunity for us to joint venture with Bionet Inc. which is one of the largest cord blood banking companies in Taiwan to explore stem cell-based clinical applications in cosmetic medicine and products.

After several years of trials, we came to the conclusion that stem cell transplant or topical stem cell culture media is quite effective locally but is at best ambiguous at the systemic level after intravenous infusion.

This phenomenon puzzled me until the summer of 2012 when the work of Dr. Carrel was brought to my attention incidentally while I was competing in the Global Launch Pad of The Booth

Business School of the University of Chicago in Beijing. Inspired by Carrel, I quickly realized that the facial skin was rejuvenated by the transdermal heterochronic parabiotic process. At the same time, based on the immortal theory of cells propose by Carrel, I was able to hypothesize that the blood plasma is like the culture media for the cells inside human body, if we can renew the plasma to a more youthful state, we might be able to reverse the aging process and extend the healthspan of human.

However, young plasma has only very limited supply and carries inevitable risks of rejection and infection. The development of anti-aging oral pills also requires a tremendous amount of money and an extended amount of time, both beyond our capacity. As a result, we decided to develop formulations composed of protein drugs approved by the FDA to create effects that mimic that of young plasma.

Our effort was made possible by modifications based on works of Irina and Michael Conboy of Berkley, U. of California and Tony Wyss-Coray of Stanford University. Eventually, we were able to engineer a formulation to simulate the effect of heterochronic parabiosis in a clinical setting which was later supported by the pioneering work of Conboys' and Dr. Dobri Kiprov in 2020.

Current protocol for our heterochronic plasma exchange is in three parts. The first is to remove harmful substances from the

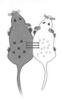

old blood, followed by addition of beneficial factors found in the young plasma. Finally, for those who are in extreme old age or in very poor health conditions, transfusion of allogeneic stem cells might be required. All of the above could be performed using one small single lumen intravenous catheter easily in an outpatient clinic setting.

During the past few years, we have performed these heterochronic plasma exchange procedures for hundreds of patients with various aging-related problems, such as: Adult-onset diabetes, Alzheimer's disease, degenerative disc joint diseases, frailty, and for the prevention of local recurrence and metastasis of solid tumors. The expectations of our patients was largely met as indicated by more than sixty percent of retention rate.

Finally, I sincerely wish the birth of this book will allow those who are interested in anti-aging technologies to gain further understanding of the developmental history, underlying mechanism, and potential clinical applications of anti-aging plasma exchange developed based on the heterochronic parabiosis experiment.

Fu-shih Pan, M.D., Ph.D.
Miraco Clinic
Taipei, Taiwan
October 5th, 2021

1. Why Is Anti-Aging Important?

Since thousands of years ago, mankind had begun the pursuit of longevity and hoping to feel and look young forever. However, to the surprise of many, modern medical society did not pay much attention to aging-related problems until the late 20 century.

Two hundred years ago, the average lifespan of humans was only 40 years. At that time, people, in general, could not live long enough to experience the aging processes.

Due to the birth of modern medicine, within the next 100 years, the average lifespan experienced a rapid rise to 55 years, which was further extended by another 25 years to reach the current life expectancy of 80 years old during the past 100 years. If this trend were able to continue, at this speed of 20 to 30 years per 100 years, some scientists project that the human life span will eventually reach the 150 years mark. However, this is unlikely to be the case.

Let us examine the age of death of United States women over the past 85 years. (Figure 1) The x-axis is the age of death, the y-axis is the number of people who died. The line on the left side is the age of death curve in 1933 and the line on the right is the age of

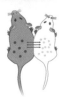

death curve in 2014. From the figure, we can see that in 1933, there were 2 peaks in the curve. The first peak occurs at birth and the other peak occurs between 70 and 90 years of age. On the other hand, there was only one peak of the 2014 age of death curve between 85 and 95. This implies that the largest increase in the average life expectancy over the past 85 years occurs due to the decrease in mortality at birth (mostly due to the advances in obstetrics and neonatal care). If we eliminate the influences of this, the actual extension in average life span was less than 15 years over the last 80 years.

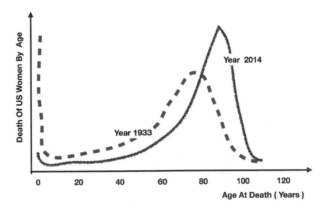

Figure 1: The distribution of death at different ages in the United States in 1933 and 2014. This indicates that the extension of the average lifespan over the last 80 years is mostly due to the decrease of mortality at birth. The average human lifespan seems to converge to the age of 90 to 100 years old. (Source: demogr.mpg.de)

Furthermore, from the changes in the spread of the above age of death curve, we also observe that the distribution of the age of death narrowed significantly over the last 80 years. This seems to imply that most people will eventually die at the same age bracket, e.g., between the age 90 and 100 as the standard of medical care continues to improve in the future; rather than extending to 150 years old as some optimistic scientists might suggest.

Should we be happy about the life extension phenomena?

According to the WHO (World Health Organization), the profile of the disease for the causes of death was very different 100 years ago. At that time (in early 1900), the most prevalent diseases and cause of death were infectious, e.g., pneumonia, influenza, tuberculosis, and gastrointestinal diseases. Over the last century, the profile of causes of death has changed dramatically. Cardiovascular, malignant tumors (e.g., cancers), and chronic obstructive pulmonary disease become the top 3 causes of death in 2018. These changes are mostly due to the advances in three important advances in medicine, namely: anesthesiology, transfusion, and antibiotics.

As people can live to an older age, aging-related diseases also begin to surface. For illustrative purposes, let us take osteoporosis as an example. Assuming the osteoporosis will occur 10 years after menopause which on average occurs at age of 50. When the

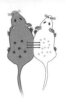

average life span is less than 50 years, only a few women can live to experience menopause and there will be very few women who can live to suffer from osteoporosis. When the average life span is between 50 and 60, there will be many people who can live to experience the menopausal symptoms, but still very few will contract the osteoporosis diseases. When the average life span passes 60, every woman will suddenly live to an old age, which allows them to experience both signs and symptoms of menopausal and osteoporosis. As a result, people will have a bone fracture from a fall and will crowd the hospital if the governing agency is not prepared ahead of time.

From the disease prevalence curve (Figure 2), we can observe that from the adult-onset Type 2 Diabetes to Cardiovascular disease, to neurodegenerative diseases, to cancer and even Covid-19, almost all of the disease incidence increases with age. The incidence of 9 out of the 10 most common diseases in developed countries, i.e., cancer, cardiovascular diseases, pneumonia, cerebrovascular incidence, diabetes, COPD, high blood pressure, nephritis, Chronic renal failure, and Cirrhosis, are in proportion to age.

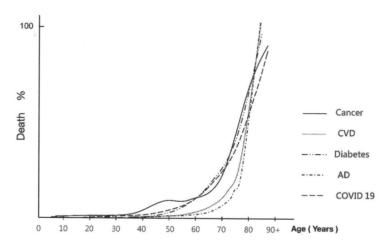

Figure 2. Prevalence of common diseases with age. The probability of contracting cardiovascular diseases, cancer diabetes, neurodegenerative diseases, and Covid-19 increases with age. As the result of increases in life span, they replaced infectious and gastrointestinal diseases to become major causes of death in developed countries,

Most of the citizens over the age of 65 are diagnosed with multiple diseases. According to a recent study in Taiwan (who has a complete medical history of her citizen under the National Health Service program), 50% of the senior were diagnosed with hypertension, 20% with Diabetes, 10% has hepatobiliary problems, and as high as 7% of this population has chronic renal diseases. This data suggests that most of the seniors are literally in the octant state of illness by definition, with further extension in life span, the length of suffering from the diseases also increases (Figure 3). It is estimated that the last 20% of our

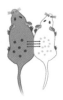

natural life span is accompanied by at least one or more chronic diseases and the unhealthy lifespan also increases steadily as the healthy life span increases.

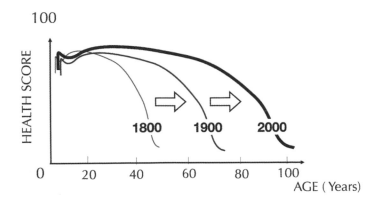

Figure 3. The relation between health and age. Over the last two centuries, the average lifespan of mankind continued to increase steadily. However, at the same time, many aging-related chronic diseases have also become more and more prevalent. This resulted also in increases in unhealthy life span.

In summary, due to the advances in medicine, the human lifespan has almost doubled over the past 200 years. However, this extension comes with the cost of increases in numerous chronic diseases and tremendous social economic burdens to society. Furthermore, it also created a vicious cycle of increases in unhealthy life span. At present, most of the seniors usually are living with and suffer from a few illnesses and hundreds of thousands of them are handicapped or bedridden, which greatly reduced the happiness that could have been achieved with the life span extension.

The general public and medical society should place a greater interest and effort to promote lifestyles in anti-aging and anti-chronic diseases. In contrary to the use of extreme therapies, e.g., respirators, ECMO (i.e., Extracorporeal Membrane Oxygenator), etc., to extend the unhealthy life span.

The goal of the next generation of medicine should be using preventive medicine or regenerative medicine to slow down or even reverse the effect of age (i.e., the aging processes) exerted in health, to maximize the length of healthspan, and preserve independent life until the very end of life (Figure 4).

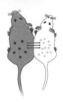

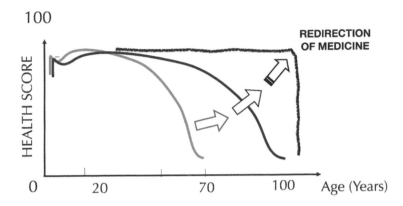

Figure 4. The true meaning of longevity is not to extend the lifespan of patients with extreme measures and technologies. Instead, we should apply preventive medicine and regenerative technologies to extend the length of the healthspan.

2. How To Live To 100 Years Of Health Span?

The first step of reaching the goal of living to one hundred years of healthspan is to understand the fundamental differences between Age and Aging.

Age is practically a unit of time. It measures the interval between the time of your birth and the current time. It is just a number. The age of a person is like the year of production of a car or a bottle of wine and bears very little information or meaning about the health condition of the person unless given further and detailed context.

Aging is the measurement of the processes or effect of time (i.e., age) on the condition of a person's state of wellness or health. It could be used to measure the conditions of a person inside the body (i.e., physiological and psychological) or outside appearance.

A young (by age) person can have an old (aging) body due to genetic or epigenetic (i.e., environmental) factors. In other words, someone can have a young birthday on the identificatIon documents while possessing poor health conditions. Similarly, someone born many years ago (aged) with a good genetic profile and healthy lifestyle can be as healthy as many young people.

Just like the age listed on the ID card is almost always different from the physiological age, the human appearance is also the same. If a person takes good care of his/her skin by avoiding sun damage, thorough cleaning, and skincare products with poor quality, and a healthy lifestyle, he/she can look very youthful until very old age, the so-called agerasia phenomena. On the other hand, we can also observe rapid aging processes occurring in the sun worshipers and lower socioeconomic populations who have no money for the care of their skin.

Another aspect of aging is psychology, the advances in neurosciences have revealed that positive thinking, relaxation, as well as the quality of sleep, all play an important role in human health. Our brain is the master of our mind and body. All physiological parameters are influenced by the brain directly or indirectly.

Many aged people have a very young mindset. Their life is driven by curiosity and continuous learning. They are actively involved in every aspect of society and are responsible for the success of many charity. Those young-at-heart citizens also possess a better health condition and look younger than their actual age. Like the mother of Tesla. On the other end of the spectrum, many senior citizens have a negative attitude about getting old. They sit around in the lobby of the nursing home without any anticipation of tomorrow. Their health condition and appearance are also older than the other group.

Based on these discussions, we can visualize the relationship between the aging process and the age as in (Figure 5). The horizontal axis is the age whose unit is time or year, the vertical axis is the degree of aging. Physical examination and

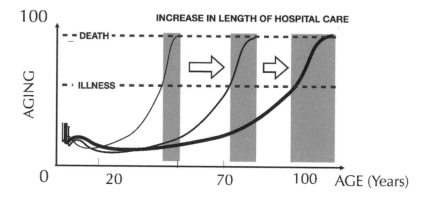

Figure 5. Relationship of the aging and age. The vertical axis represents the degree of aging and the horizontal axis indicates the age of time in years.

physiological measurements suggest that most people are healthy before the age of 50, however, this will change rapidly

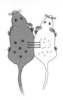

after this. The rate of aging slowly increases with time. The horizontal dash line in the middle of the figure represents the threshold of diseases and the end of the healthspan.

After the end of healthspan, the rate of aging varies greatly between patients of similar diseases. If adequate medical care were available and the patient was willing to modify their inappropriate lifestyle accordingly, then the rate of disease progression might be managed and developed at a slow rate. On the contrary, if the patient were not able to receive proper medical care or continued on a poor lifestyle, the disease might progress rapidly and lead to a need for hospitalization or intensive care. Ironically, the better the medical care actually might result in a long unhealthy life span. To enjoy a longer healthspan, anti-aging lifestyle and intervention are therefore of utmost importance.

The rate of aging varies greatly between individuals. (Figure 6) Numerous factors have been proposed to account for the process of aging. These include chronic inflammation, fibrosis, telomere shortening, free radicals, cellular senescence, etc., just to name a few. However, there are only two major categories, i.e., genetics and epigenetic. The genetics factors are parental and pre-programmed while the epigenetic factors are environmental factors that occurred after fertilization.

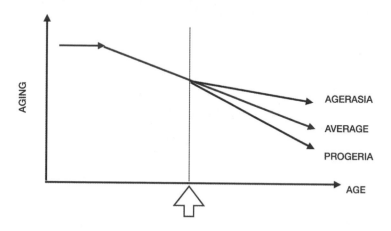

Figure 6. The rate of aging varies greatly among different individuals. Under similar environments and lifestyles, some people aged gracefully as an agerasia; while the others might age rapidly as in the case of progeria.

The genetic principle is evident from the fact that given the same lifestyle and environment, the identical twins might have aged similarly but other individuals will most likely have aged at different rates. On the other hand, identical twins who were brought up in a different environment aged differently also revealed the importance of epigenetic factors.

The purpose of anti-aging medicine or rejuvenation medicine is to slow down or stop the aging processes and reverse the effects caused by it. (Figure 7) Since aging is the number one cause of all diseases in developed countries, anti-aging medicine will be able to reverse the progression of aging-related diseases, e.g., coronary artery disease, adult-onset diabetes, etc. As a result, people might be able to live longer with a shorter unhealthy life span both inside and outside the body.

The advances in the past several decades in anti-aging medicine are mostly focused on studying the positive effects of a healthy lifestyle in delaying the aging processes; The scientific and medical community, however, still facing a shortage of technologies that might be applied to reversing the aging-related disease conditions (i.e., rejuvenation medicine).

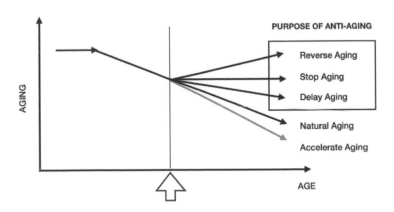

Figure 7. Anti-aging medicine and aging reversal. The goal of anti-aging medicine is to apply medical intervention to delay, stop, and reverse the process of aging.

3. How To Reverse The Aging Processes?

Just like a citizen is the smallest unit of a nation, the smallest unit of the human body is the cell. Together with the ground substances, the cells form various types of tissues which are further integrated into different organs. Several organs might work together to become a system that carries one of the vital functions required by our body to sustain our life, e.g., cardiovascular, pulmonary, renal, ...etc.

Just like the body is separated from the outside environment by the skin and is equipped with various organs inside, the cell also contains many miniature organs, called organelles, e.g., Golgi body, mitochondria, endoplasmic reticulum, inside of its membrane, i.e., a lipid-bilayer surface that separates the inside of the cell (i.e., cytosol) from the outside environment (i.e., interstitial space).

With time, microscopically, the organelles become dysfunctional from wear and tear, which resulted in aging at the cellular level. This will then advance to the aging at the tissue, the organ, and the system level. (Figure 8) When the dysfunction is irreversible, the diseases occur and progress to result in system failure if left unattended. When three or more of the systems

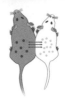

fail to carry out normal functions our life will usually enter the final stage and soon be terminated.

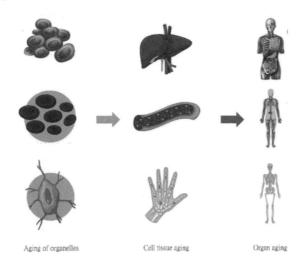

Aging of organelles   Cell tissue aging   Organ aging

Figure 8. The relationship between the aging of cellular organelles and the human body. As time went by, the organelles in the cell also gradually aged. This will result in aging at the cellular, tissue, organ, and system levels. As a result, the function of the body begins to deteriorate and aging-related degenerative disease occurs.

Contrary to the above bottom-up (i.e., microscopic) viewpoint, we can also examine the aging process in a top-down fashion. Macroscopically, the human body is constantly in an equilibrium and homeostasis state between the force of destruction and force of reconstruction. Assuming the lifestyle, mental stress, and environmental factors are in a constant state, then the force of destruction will also be a constant. In this case, the wellness state or the health condition may be solely determined by the force of reconstruction.

If the force of destruction is less than the force of reconstruction, the damages caused by the destruction will be repaired efficiently in a timely manner, there would not be any residual damages (Figure 9). This is what happens when the person is young and is called the youthful state.

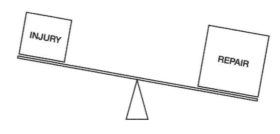

INJURY < REPAIR = YOUTH

Figure. 9. State of youthfulness. Our body is constantly influenced by the force of destruction and reconstruction. When the force of reconstruction is larger than that of the destruction, everything is maintained in optimal conditions and functions properly. This is called the state of youthfulness.

On the other hand, when the force of reconstruction is less than the rate of destruction, there will be some residual damages that might not be repaired and restored on time, as the trauma continues and the damaged tissues gradually accumulate, the scarring or permanent injuries resulting (Figure 10). This condition usually occurs when the subjects grow older and are in the state of aging.

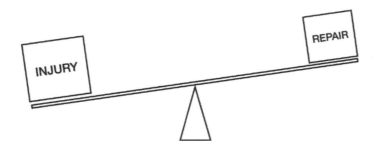

INJURY > REPAIR = AGING

Figure 10. When the force of destruction exceeds the force of reconstruction. There will be some residual defects left un-repaired after each traumatic event, which is the state of aging.

Many methods might decrease the speed of destruction. For example, a healthy diet e.g. low in sugar and unsaturated fatty acids, avoidance of processed food products (e.g., nitric oxides from smoke preserved food), and environmental pollutions (e.g., PM2.5 particles, tar of cigarette smoking, and intense electromagnetic radiations), as well as the reduction in daily stress by positive thinking, mediation, etc.. All of these might reduce the rate of destruction both inside and outside of our bodies.

There are also effective means that can enhance the rate of reconstruction in the human body, namely, nutrition and exercise. The nutrients are materials and tools required for the body to carry out necessary reconstruction processes. These are quite different from nutrition that produces energy, i.e., calories, for daily activities. Lack of proper nutrition can delay the wound healing process while proper nutrition can facilitate and accelerate the repair. Exercise is also important for maintaining our body's repair capacity. As exercise can increase circulation which is like the transportation system. A healthy circulatory system can transport the oxygen, nutrients, and cells to the site of injury to repair damaged tissues.

All of the above-mentioned methods are popular topics frequently being addressed and promoted in the senior community. Together they could be categorized as Lifestyle Medicine (Figure 11). The characteristics of these methods are

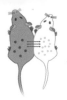

low entry barriers (do not require lots of money or extensive professional assistance) and extremely high exit criteria (i.e., strongly rely upon one's own will to continue the treatment for a long time before significant effects could be observed). Although these lifestyle changes were all proven effective, it is extremely difficult to ask a senior person to change his/her lifestyle or habits, e.g., smoking, mindset, or addiction to sweets, etc. This left many spaces for the practice of anti-aging medicine.

There were numerous products and services available in the market for the baby boomer generation. The products range from supplements to home exercise machines to APP for the creation of a healthy lifestyle, the services range from the spa, chiropractor, aromatherapy, to both non-invasive and invasive anti-aging medicine. Although all of these have their own beliefs and niche markets in different parts of the world, the scientific and medical community has long been lacking any clinical guidelines.

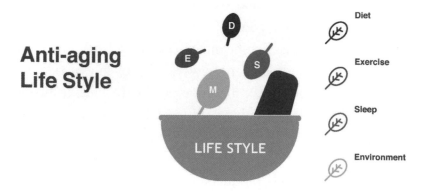

Figure 11. A person can reduce the force of destruction by a healthy diet, clean environment, and relaxation; while the force of reconstruction might be reinforced by adequate nutrition and exercises. However, all of these involve lifestyle change and are very difficult for most people to execute for a prolonged time.

Here, we would like to limit our scope of anti-aging medicine to interventions (not included in the lifestyle medicine) that might counteract the effect of age by increasing repair capacity in our bodies.

In 2015, Nature published a news article which picked the top 6 anti-aging technologies that might eventually be translated into clinical practice. These also set a standard for developing new technologies in the future to compare with in terms of the scientific and clinical evidence that are required to gather.

The first method on Nature's 2015 list is caloric restriction. This is arguably the most studied anti-aging method. The data ranging from the laboratory mice to the primate suggested that animals can extend their life span by 15% to 30% of their calorie intakes were reduced by 30%. Although there were no human trials, judging from the popularity of the intermittent fasting programs, this method is proven to be acceptable to the general public. As a result, regardless of the outcome of studies addressing the amount of lifespan extension that could be achieved, this is already the front runner among all anti-aging methods.

Second on Nature's list is Resveratrol, a chemical found in red wine. Resveratrol has been widely studied in laboratory animals, it can trigger the mTOR (i.e., mammalian Target Of Rapamycin) pathway and stimulate the autophagy (i.e., self-eating) process which plays a crucial role in the prevention of cellular aging. However, to receive enough quantity of resveratrol, one will need to consume liters of red wine. Therefore, some supplement companies have developed and marketed products made of grape seeds. Large scale clinical trial on the efficacy of resveratrol in lifespan extension is still not available.

The next on the list is Rapamycin which is an antibiotic first discovered in the earth of Easter Island. Like resveratrol, rapamycin can stimulate the autophagy process to slow down or reverse cellular aging, however, its application is discouraged due to the immunosuppressive side effects to the human.

Every cell has a nucleus that contains DNA molecules. The DNA molecule is where the code of genetics is located and is responsible for the propagation of human life. The DNA is composed of a sequence of purines and pyrimidines, i.e., Adenine, Thymine, Guanine, Cytosine.

At the end of the DNA molecule, there is a long repeating sequence of bases called the telomere. It acts as the protection of the main body of the DNA which contains genetic information. This is like the plastic caps at the end of each shoelace. It was found in the 1990s that the length of this sequence is in direct proportion to the age of the cell by Elizabeth Blackburn who was awarded the Nobel Prize in Physiology and Medicine in 2012.

Related to telomere there is an RNA and protein complex called Telomerase, which can extend the length of the telomere. Since the telomere of each cell is shortened with each cell division, the elongation of the telomere will allow the cell to divide more times which, in theory, implies a longer life span of the cell. Although telomerase was included in the shortlist of potential rejuvenation methods chosen by Nature, these are limited to animal experiments. Since telomerase extends the length of telomeres, some might think of it as changing the "height" of someone without actually changing their function. Its clinical indications are under intense discussion.

When Nature published its potential list of clinical anti-aging technologies in 2015, stem cells were at the central stage of biological science. The stem cell is one of the 4 categories of cells (i.e., sperm/oocyte, their precursor cells, somatic cells, somatic stem cells) that resides in the human body. It is responsible for the repair of damaged tissues. Since anti-aging is to increase the repair capacity of the body, almost all scientists expect that the advances in stem cell science will allow scientists and doctors to repair, rejuvenate, and regenerate any damaged tissues and organs in the future. According to the Principles of Regenerative Medicine declared in 1992, stem cells form the central triad with the scaffold and the cytokines, many scientists are working on optimizing the formulation to produce artificial tissues and organs to replace the damaged ones. However, this approach is only valid locally in practice, and is difficult to apply at a systemic level.

The last method on Nature's list of anti-aging methods is the young blood. Both in the history of east and west, there are many stories that value the bright red blood as the origin of life and vitality. There are also many stories regarding implementing this mysterious fluid to delay and or reverse the aging processes. In China Taoism, the alchemist had practiced the Principle of Cai-yin-bu-yang (i.e., which means having intercourse with young women to absorb their youth power). In the west there are stories of Erzsébet Báthory in Hungary and vampire stories from the Eastern Romania region, describing the immortality that could be achieved by ingestion of the bright red blood.

Because transfusion is a FDA approved procedure which is part of standard of care for many decades, there is a surge of interest in transfusion of blood from young donors (as a shortcut) to meet the urgent need of aging reversal by the large number of baby boomers entering age of 60's and beyond. Although this concept has attracted large interest from the public and reporters from almost all major media, the anti-aging effect of young blood transfusion on the aging body is yet to be proven.

Unlike the convalescent plasma therapy for the Covid-19, FDA had issued a warning regarding the efficacy of this treatment in 2019. However, the interest remains and continues to grow.

4. What Is Stem Cell ?

Human development begins with the entrance of sperm of father into the egg of mother, together they form a cell which is called the zygote. After the zygote embedded in the endometrium of the uterus, the cell begins to divide from one to two, to four, and eight cells, …, to form a small aggregate of cells called the inner mass. Until this time, each of the cells has the capacity to grow and form an individual. These cells are capable of differentiating into any cell type, i.e., totipotent.

As the development continues with further cell divisions, the differentiation capacity of the cells decreased to multiple cell types limited to one of the three germ layers, namely the ectoderm, the mesoderm, and the endoderm. In other words, the differentiation capacity of the cells in the embryo decreases as the number of the cells increases before the birth of the fetus.

After the birth, our body has only 4 types of cells, i.e., sperm or oocyte, precursor cell of sperm/oocyte, somatic cell, and adult stem cell. The sperm and eggs as well as their precursor cells, which are called spermatozoa and oocyte, are responsible for the reproduction. The somatic cells are responsible for the routine works of the human body, and the precursor cells of Somali cells, which are called the adult stem cells and reside in each major organ, are responsible for the repair of injured tissues.

There are no embryonic cells in the human body after birth, as the result, transplantation of which is probably unnecessary and might impose un-predictable risk on the recipient.

The adult stem cells residing in each organ are usually in a dormant stage; when the tissues of the organ experience auto trauma or become defected from normal wear and tear, the adjacent somatic cells will release cytokines to activate the adult stem cell. The activated adult stem cell will divide into two separate cells. (Figure 12)

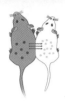

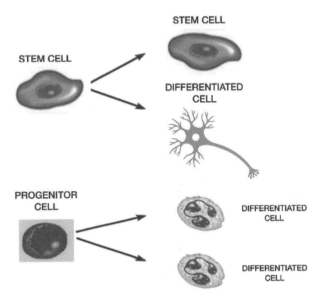

Figure 12. Division of stem cells, When the tissue is damaged, the adult stem cell at the adjacent location will be activated and begin to divide into two different cells. One is exactly like itself, i.e. an adult stem cell, the other will become a precursor cell of a somatic cell, also called the progenitor cell.

One is identical to itself, and the other will become the precursor cell of a somatic cell, i.e., progenitor cell. It is able to differentiate into a somatic cell to fill the vacancy created by the injuries.

Although the origin of adult stem cells is ambiguous, their role in replacing injured cells and damaged tissues have achieved a general consensus in all disciplines of regenerative medicine.

5. How To Improve Repair Capacity Of Stem Cell?

The main purpose of anti-aging medicine is to increase the repair capacity of the human body. Since the adult stem cells are the cell types responsible for the repair; anti-aging medicine could be considered to improve repair capacity of the human body by increasing the number or function of the adult stem cell.

Before the age of 50, the number of adult stem cells and their function are usually within the normal range. After the age of 50, both inside and outside of the cell would have accumulated many pollutants. the function of the stem cell begins to decrease. Eventually, the stem cell might become apoptotic, i.e., cell death, and the number of stem cells will decrease.

Generally speaking, the repair capacity of the human body begins to decrease after 50 years of age, by the time of 80 to 90 years old, the number of the stem cells in the tissues are less than 30% as compared to the young people (Figure 13), while their function is also only a portion of their younger counterparts.

In order to slow down the aging processes, we have to slow down the rates of the loss of stem cells and the decay of their functions.

In order to reverse the aging process, we have to increase the number of the stem cells and increase their function to increase the repair capacity of the human body.

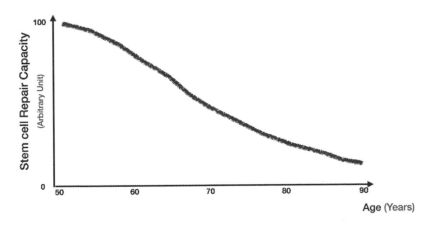

Figure 13. The decrease of the number of stem cells after the age of 50. The calculation is based on a population model.

Let us examine another aging model which is more clinically relevant (Figure 14). In this model, the rectangular on the left side represents a young human body, while the left side represents an aging human body. In the model, the small cased "c" represents a younger cell which usually is smaller in size, the capital "C" represents an older cell which is usually larger in size.

The small circle "∘ " represents various nutrient molecules, and

43

the little "★" represents growth factors and cytokines that might

stimulate and activate the somatic cell and adult stem cell. The arrow pointing towards the right side indicates the aging process which is an oxidative process. Finally, the arrow pointing towards the left side indicates the rejuvenation process which is a reduction process.

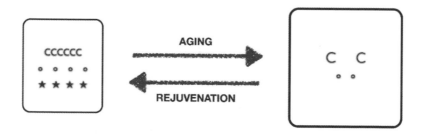

Figure 14. A simple model for anti-aging. The rounded square on the left represents tissue in a young person, while the left side represents that of an older person.

It can be seen from this model that there are more cells in the young human body; because the absorption capacity is better, the nutrition is more sufficient; and because of development and growth, the concentration of cytokines and hormones in the body is also higher.

The right side of the model represents an elderly human body, we can see that the number of cells is relatively small; due to insufficient gastrointestinal absorption, nutrition might not be enough; the most important thing is that there are basically not many cytokines and hormones in the elderly body to awake the stem cells in the elderly. This further leads to a significant reduction in the repair function of stem cells.

If you want to reverse aging, you must improve the repairing power of stem cells, that is, increase the number and function of stem cells. The greater the number of stem cells in an organ, or the better the function of stem cells, the better the bodies can repair or regenerate itself.

How to increase the number of stem cells?

After a person is born, the stem cells in the organ are usually in a dormant state, and the number will not increase. If you want to increase the number of stem cells, you can only implant stem cells from outside the body. (Figure 15)

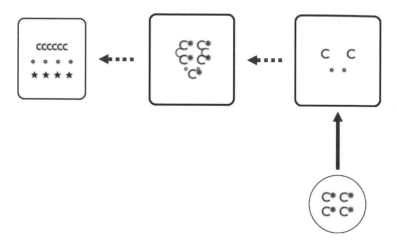

Figure 15. Diagram of stem cell transplantation. After the human body is born, the stem cells in the organs are usually in a dormant state, and the number will not increase. If the number of cells is to be increased, stem cells can only be implanted into the body from outside the body.

Stem cells used in clinics and laboratories have three major sources: autologous, allogeneic and xenogeneic. (Figure 16)

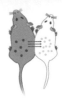

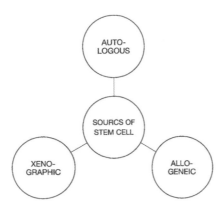

Figure 16. The source of stem cells. Stem cells used for culture have three major sources: autologous (the recipient himself), allogeneic (another person), and xenographic (animal).

Autologous stem cells represent stem cells extracted from one's own internal organs or tissues. Its advantage is that it has the same genes of other cells in the body and will not be attacked by the immune system, as the result, it will not induce rejection or other adverse reactions and the survival rate of the transplanted cells is high. The disadvantages of the autologous stem cells are as follows, in general, people who need to improve their repair ability are older, so their stem cells are older and their number in the tissue is relatively small, so it is difficult to harvest and cultivate. Even if the laboratory can extract their stem cells from the tissues of the elderly and cultured them successfully, after the implantation, the repair function is worse than that of the young stem cells.

In 2006, Professor Shinya Yamanaka of Plastic Surgery at Kyoto University in Japan developed the Induced Pluripotent Stem (IPS) Cell technology, which uses four different transcription factors: Oct4, Sox2, c-Myc and Klf4, to restore adult somatic cells (i.e., fibroblast) back to the state of embryonic stem cells. Although Professor Yamanaka won the 2012 Nobel Prize in Medicine for this important research, however, due to the oncogenic potential of the c-Myc gene, there are safety concerns in the clinical settings and still require a lot of studies before IPS could be translated into clinical settings.

The second source of stem cells is adult stem cells obtained from other people's bodies. Because stem cells are not fully differentiated, they will not induce strong rejection after transplantation. However, in the long run, they will still be rejected by the recipient's own immune system and cannot survive forever. The advantage of allogeneic stem cells is that the donors are usually very young, once these young stem cells enter the body, they will exert their repair capacity rapidly and achieve better effects in the short term as compare to the stem cell from an old donor.

The third source of stem cells is xerographic stem cells from animals. The vitality of animal stem cells is much stronger than

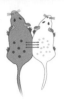

that of human stem cells. Unfortunately, it also could induce a strong rejection and immune response in the human body, so the survival rate is lowest among the three common sources. Although xenogeneic stem cells are easily available and inexpensive, the risk of transplantation is relatively high. There are only a few clinics in Switzerland and Germany still engaged in clinical work related to xenographic stem cells transplant.

How to improve the function of stem cells?

In addition to increasing the number of stem cells in the body through stem cell transplantation, we can also use nutrition and exercise to improve the function of stem cells and repair ability in the body. Fasting or intermittent fasting and exercise are important parts of lifestyle medicine. Although it does not seem to cost much and seems to be easily achieved, however, it is extremely difficult to maintain these for a long time. Clinically, successful cases are relatively rare.

The function of stem cells can also be enhanced by various growth hormones, such as growth hormones and androgen or estrogen. (Figure 17) However, these drugs each have their side effects. Growth hormones can cause insulin resistance and increase in blood glucose. It may also cause edema of the joints and reduce patient's daily activity. Male or female hormones could mildly increase the risk of some form of cancers (i.e., those with hormonal receptors). It is recommended to take various hormonal therapy only periodically, and is not an ideal anti-aging method.

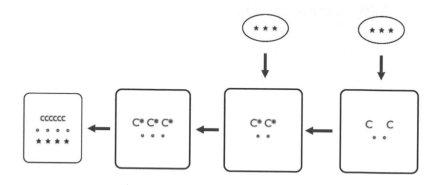

Figure 17. Growth hormone enhances stem cell function. To enhance the function of stem cells in the body and the body's repair ability, stem cell transplantation, balanced nutrition and exercise can all be used.

Based on the effects exert on the repair capacity of the stem cell, the anti-aging options proposed by the Nature in 2015 can be divided into two categories: stem cell transplantation is to increase repair capacity by increase the number of stem cells; calorie restriction (various fasting program included), resveratrol, rapamycin, and young blood increase the repair power of stem cells by activating them with biological and chemical factors. As for telomerase, it is a tool to increase the

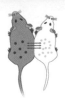

number of divisions that could be performed by the stem cells and might increase the repair capacity indirectly.

6. How Good Is The Effect Of Stem Cell Therapy?

For the past few decades, after continuous efforts of cross disciplined physicians and scientists, a number of clinical trials related to anti-aging medicine have been completed. Although everyone has reached a consensus on improving the repairing power of stem cells to fight aging, however, there is still a lot of controversy as to how to improve the repairing power of stem cells clinically.

We can use a 2 by 2 Table to examine the current status of applications of the stem cells in anti-aging related clinical medicine. (Figure 18)

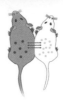

STEM CELL THERAPIES	LOCAL INJECTION (Regenerative Medicine)	SYSTEMIC INFUSION (Rejuvenation Medicine)
NUMBER (Stem Cell Transplant)	1	2
FUNCTION (Stem Cell Activation)	3	4

** Facial (Anti-aging Skincare)

Figure 18. The matrix to be used for the assessment of the clinical use of stem cells in anti-aging medicine.

The first column shows two ways to improve the repair capacity of stem cells. The first is to increase the number of stem cells by stem cell transplantation, and the second is to enhance the function of stem cells by hormones and cytokines that might activate the stem cell function.

The first row shows the two major clinical applications of stem cells. The first is local treatment usually carried by direct injection (i.e., local treatments for organs is generally called regenerative medicine; while local treatment for facial skin is generally called anti-aging treatments or products). The second is systemic treatment usually carried out by intravenous or intramuscular or subcutaneous injection. The goal is to delay and to stop the aging processes, and eventually reverse the aging effect of the entire body and is the focus of the remainder of this book.

Local stem cell transplant is to inject stem cells directly into the aging organ. In Europe and the United States, doctors have been injecting bone marrow stem cells, adipose stem cells or allogeneic umbilical cord stem cells cultured in the laboratory into the necrotic heart tissue due to myocardial infarction to promote the regeneration of heart muscle cells. In Asia, doctors also have been injecting stem cells into the necrotic brain tissue due to stroke to promote the regeneration of nerve cells in the brain. Orthopedic doctors also have been injecting stem cells into the joints, which are worn out due to weight bearing, to promote regeneration of the cartilage.

Local stem cell transplants are also quite popular in aesthetic medicine. Since the adipose-derived stem cells were isolated in 2002, plastic surgeons or aesthetic medical doctors are able to separate ADSC (i.e., Adipose Derived Stem Cells) from the aspirate of liposuction procedure and injected them back into the skin of the face or hands, to remove the wrinkles (Figure 19) or to lighten up the color of the skin (Figure 20). They also inject ADSC into the atrophic hair follicles on the scalp to promote regeneration of hair follicles (Figure 21) (Figure 22) for the

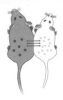

treatment of androgenic alopecia or baldness as the result of burn scars or trauma.

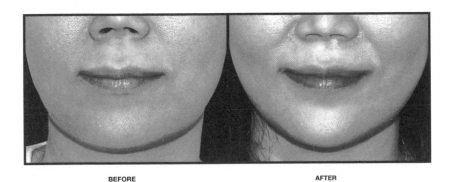

BEFORE AFTER

Figure 19. The wrinkle removal effect of adipose stem cell injection on the face.

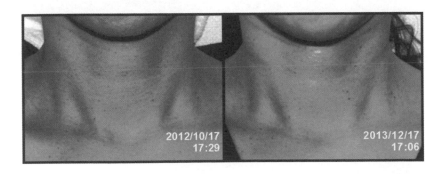

2012/10/17 17:29   2013/12/17 17:06

Figure 20. The whitening effect of adipose stem cell injection on the skin of the neck.

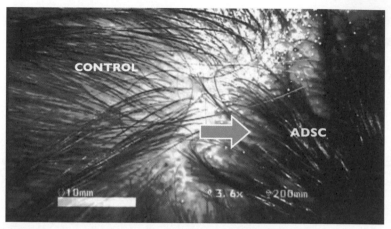

Figure 21. The regenerative effect of adipose stem cell injection on the atrophic hair follicle. The figure shows an increase in hair diameter and density at the injection site (right lower corner which is marked as ADSC) as compared to the non-injected sites (left upper corner which is marked as control).

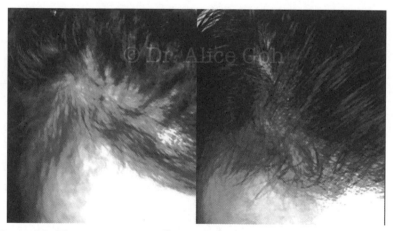

Figure 22. The regenerative effect of atrophic hair follicles injected with adipose derived stem cells.

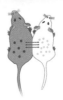

For safety and quality assurance reasons, regulatory organs usually restrict the separation of adipose stem cells to be completed in the operating room. This will require participation of a surgeon, well trained nursing staff, specially trained laboratory technicians, etc. and a long time in the operation room. Therefore, the cost is very high for the procedure and the procedure could not be popularized despite the excellent results of these aesthetics procedures.

Due to the high cost of regenerative medicine, some biotech companies began to develop technologies of using conditioned medium (i.e., media collected from cell culture) of stem cell to activate stem cells in the body, hoping to replace the expensive stem cell transplantation for applications of regenerative medicine for the heart, joints, skin, and hair follicles. Because of the low cost and good effect, it is more acceptable to the market. This also became the most successful and mature business model in the anti-aging industry.

There are generally only two ways for systemic stem cell transplantation. One is to inject stem cells directly into each major organ. The other is to infuse the stem cells into the patient's body via intravenous catheter.

If direct injection is used, in order to achieve a systemic anti-aging effect, the client must receive general anesthesia to allow the physician to inject cultured stem cells directly into the heart, lungs, liver and other important organs; this method has a high risk and obviously none of the patient is willing to accept such therapy.

As early as 1992, scientists at the University of Chicago already tried to use arterial angiography to eliminate the need of direct injection.However, because of the risk of embolism and tissue necrosis resulted in, it could not be applied clinically.

In general, the concept of increasing the number of stem cells by intravenous infusion is acceptable to most of the people seeking systemic anti-aging effects. The infused stem cells will first be returned to the right atrium and right ventricle after the intravenous infusion. They will then be ejected to the lungs, passing through the capillaries for oxygenation before traveling back to the left heart, where they will again be ejected and distributed to the rest of the body via the arterial vascular system.

The diameter of stem cells is approximately three to five times larger than that of an ordinary cell. As a result, they will usually get stuck in the capillaries of the lungs, and cannot return to the left atrium and could never reach the other organs in the body.

Although intravenous infusion of stem cells had been practiced for a long time, their systemic anti-aging effect could therefore never be clearly documented.

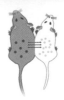

There are many stem cell companies and clinics around the world, who promote the use of stem cell infusion to delay aging and to treat various degenerative diseases. Because most of them have failed to achieve significant systemic anti-aging effects, and could not fulfill the expectation of their clients, resulting in many consumer disputes. As a result, the FDA has issued warnings against the use of stem cells for the purpose of systemic anti-aging.

Due to the difficulty of stem cells to bypass the pulmonary capillary network, the use of stem cell activation technology to increase the repair function became the only feasible method for achieving systemic anti-aging effect.

Different from stem cell transplantation, hormones and cytokines can be quickly distributed all over the body after being intravenously infused to enhance the function of stem cells residing in the organs of the entire body. However, the cost of these cytokines and hormones are very high, and the half-life of these factors and hormones are very short and require frequent infusion. Almost no one can afford the cumulative price and inconvenience required by such a program.

The stem cell treatment matrix (Figure 23) represents the current strategies and tactics regarding how to apply stem cells to increase the repair capacity of the human body by either repairing local damaged tissues or systemic anti-aging effects.

RESULT OF STEM CELL THERAPY	LOCAL INJECTION (Regenerative Medicine)	SYSTEMIC INFUSION (Rejuvenation Medicine)
NUMBER (Stem Cell Transplant)	GOOD	CONFLICTING
FUNCTION (Stem Cell Activation)	GOOD	FAIR

** Facial (Anti-aging Skincare)

Figure 23. The repair effect of stem cell activation technology. The stem cell treatment matrix shows that the use of stem cell activation technology to repair locally damaged tissues is quite effective and highly accepted, and the use of stem cell transplantation to repair damaged tissues is also effective, but the acceptance is low due to the relatively high price.

The matrix shows that the use of stem cell transplantation to repair damaged tissues has a good effect, but due to the high price, the acceptance is low; the result of using stem cell activation technology to repair locally damaged tissues is also good, and is more affordable, and the acceptance rate is higher.

The use of stem cell transplantation for systemic anti-aging is very limited. This is due to the larger size of most stem cells injected through the vein. They are usually accumulated in the capillaries of the lungs and cannot reach the whole body. Direct injection of stem cells into every vital organ is feasible theoretically, however, has never been performed. As of the use of stem cell activation by various hormones and cytokines, it is limited by the extremely high price.

Although the doctors and scientists have always been very positive regarding the use of stem cells to enhance the body's repair ability and to reverse the effects of aging, the progress in anti-aging medicine, especially in the field of systemic anti-aging, is actually very limited.

7. Who Is Dr. Carrel?

One of the most talented and contributors in the field of modern surgery should be the winner of the Nobel Prize in Physiology and Medicine in 1912, Dr. Alexis Carrel from France. (Figure 24)

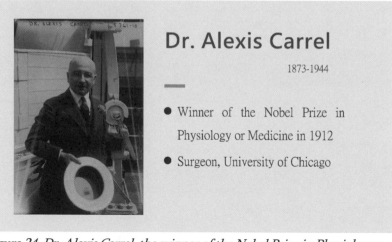

Figure 24. Dr. Alexis Carrel, the winner of the Nobel Prize in Physiology and Medicine in 1912. (Source: nobelprize.org)

Dr. Carrel was born in Lyon, France in 1873. When he was studying medicine at the University of Lyon in France in 1894, the French President Marie François Sadi Carnot was shot and

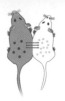

killed. His blood vessels in the liver were injured and the group of doctors responsible for rescuing him failed to repair the blood vessels. The group doctors were helpless and the president died of bleeding. Dr. Carrel, who was still a student, observed the whole situation and was determined to develop surgical techniques to repair injured blood vessels.

Due to Dr. Carrel's personal talent and hard work, by referring to the method used by tailors to sew hollow cloth strips, he soon developed the "three-point vascular suture technique", which has been used by surgeons to this day, and became the father of vascular surgery.

Due to the complicated relationship between the factions of the French Academy of Medicine, Carrel could not find a proper job in France after graduation, and was unable to continue his research. He decided to leave France and travel to the United States via Canada to seek opportunities for further career development. Eventually, he found a job as a researcher in the Hull Laboratory of School of Medicine at the University of Chicago. He then started his brilliant career in the history of modern surgery.

During his time of working at the Medical School of The University of Chicago, he performed numerous researches and developed many applications of his vascular suture technique. Under the guidance of Professor Stewart, carried worked with

Charles Claude Guthrie to perform many interesting animal experiments, such as: blood vessel transplantation, organ transplantation, limb transplantation, and even head transplantation. Dr. Carrel published a total of 29 papers at the University of Chicago, laid down the foundation for cardiovascular and organ transplant surgery for the future.

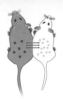

8. What Is Heterochronic Parabiosis?

Perhaps when Dr. Carrel was at the University of Chicago, he already had a preliminary idea for anti-aging medicine in the future, so he carried out an interesting experiment which was called Heterochronic Parabiosis (Hetero: different, Chronic: age, Para: common, Biosis: life).

After anesthesia, Carrel connected the frank skin of an old mouse and a young mouse, allowing them to establish a blood circulation system which allows them to share the blood of each other (Figure 25). The paired animals were sacrificed in a few weeks. He examined the internal organs of the two mice under a microscope; it turned out that the organs of the old mice became younger, while the organs of the young mice became old.

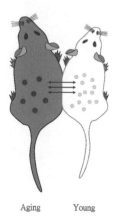

Aging   Young

Figure 25. Siamese experiment of two mice called Heterochronic Parabiosis.
Dr. Carrel connected the back skin of the old mouse and the young mouse,
allowing for sharing each other's blood; five weeks later, he found that the
organs of the old mice were getting younger, while the organs of the young
rats were getting old.

This famous conjoined animal experiment for young and old is
the first method in human history that has been proven to
reverse aging. At that time, and even now, it was a terrifying
experiment!

It's a pity that people can't be connected ethically, and can't be
done clinically!

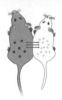

Regarding the underlying mechanism of aging reversal in the old animal of the old-young pair, most of the scientists believe it is due to the rejuvenation effects of youthful factors composed in the blood of the young animal of the old-young pair.

Because human conjoining is clinically impossible, almost all of the translational efforts of doctors and scientists were focused on separating these youthful factors from the young blood and then injecting these anti-aging ingredients into the aging body by intravenous or intramuscular route, to achieve the purpose of aging reversal.

After Dr. Carrel left the University of Chicago, he worked as a researcher at the newly established Rockefeller University and set up a laboratory to find substances in young animals that can keep the cells in the culture staying young forever.

Dr. Carrel first took out the heart of the chicken and cultured it in a petri dish. Under normal circumstances, the heart cells of chickens can only survive for a few weeks. However, Dr. Carrel used a special juice prepared by a unique formula of smashing chicken embryos as well as addition of specific amino acids and chemicals, to keep the cultured chicken heart cells alive in a petri dish continuously from 1916 for 34 years with the help of his assistant. (Figure 26) Based on this experimental result, Carrel came to a conclusion that the cells could be kept immortal should they receive proper nutrition at certain intervals and proposed his famous "The Cell Is Immortal" theory.

Dr. Carrel returned to France after retired from Rockefeller University in 1940. This experiment was forced to stop. His many years of experiments could not be continued, which is a great loss in the history of anti-aging medicine.

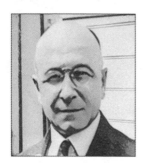

THE CELL IS IMMORTAL.

" It is merely the fluid in which it floats which degenerates. Renew this fluid at intervals, give the cells something on which to feed and, so far as we know, the pulsation of life may go on forever ... "

Alexis Carrel

Figure 26. Dr. Carrel's chicken embryo experiment. Beginning in 1916, Dr. Carrel used his unique chicken embryo juice formula to successfully cultivate chicken heart cells in a petri dish for more than 30 years.

Because humans cannot be connected clinically, and Dr. Carrel returned to France in the late World War II, he was suspected of being a supporter of the Nazi government, his heterochronic parabiosis experiments gradually became forgotten by the mainstream scientists and physicians. Only a few European physicians, including himself, undaunted by difficulties continued to develop methods to translate the heterochronic parabiosis experiments to clinical medicine.

At that time, Dr. Carrel's Heterochronic Parabiosis experiment attracted the attention of Dr. Paul Niehans, who became the founder of the famous La Prairie therapy. (Figure 27)

Dr. Niehans is a Swiss surgeon, graduated from the Bern Medical College in Switzerland, and then trained as a resident in Zurich. He was a well-known surgeon for glandular surgery of the head and neck at that time.

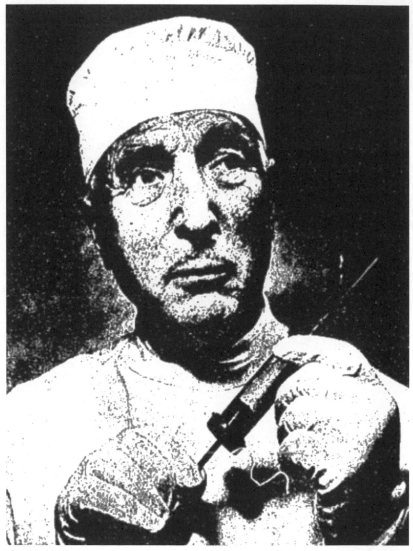

Figure 27. Dr. Paul Niehans, the founder of the famous La Prairie Live Cell Therapy.

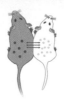

There is a pair of glandular structures called the thyroid gland in the middle of the neck, which secretes thyroid hormones which are necessary for life. Within the thyroid gland, there is a pair of tiny glands like a small bean called the parathyroid gland. The main function of the parathyroid gland is to secrete parathyroid hormone, which is responsible for maintaining the balance of calcium in the body. If the parathyroid gland is accidentally removed during thyroid surgery, calcium ions level in the blood will drop and the patient will have spasms. If not treated immediately, it may lead to death due to inability to breathe.

Once when Dr. Niehans was outside the hospital, in a place without an operating room, he encountered a young female patient who's parathyroid was accidentally removed. In the critical moment, Dr. Niehans was inspired by Dr. Carrel's Heterochronic Parabiosis experiment and thought about the concept of "like replaces alike". Since there happened to be a near term pregnant ewe around, he took out the fetus of the ewe, separated the parathyroid gland from the fetus, pulverized it into a mushy liquid, and injected it into the young lady whose parathyroid was accidentally removed.

Amazingly, the patient recovered immediately and she continued to survive for the rest of her life with this therapy without any sequelae. After having this successful case, Dr. Niehans started a xenogeneic Heterochronic Parabiosis treatment program of replacing what was missing with the extracts of the counterparts of fetal animals.

The young tissue used by Dr. Niehans comes from black sheep in the Alps, so he established Clinique La Prairie in Montreux, where the black sheep was produced, and specialized in various therapies using fetal cells of sheep.

Although Dr. Niehans treatment is not recognized by mainstream medicine and scientists, it gradually became famous probably due to good clinical results. It has attracted many celebrities in the western world to accept this type of treatment, i.e., using sheep fetal extract to treat various intractable diseases. The patients of La Prairie Therapy invented by Dr. Niehans include famous people in almost all fields of Western world, including: religious leaders: Pope Pius XII; politicians: British Prime Minister Churchill, South African President Mandela, and movie stars: Charlie Chaplin, Elisabeth Taylor, and many others, are his clients (Figure 28).

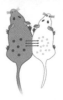

9. What Is Placenta Extract ?

In addition to Switzerland and Germany in the West, a Japanese company called Laennec was established in 1970 which applied Dr. Carrel's concept of heterochronic parabiosis therapy to develop biological agents for the treatment of liver-related diseases; Laennec and another company called Melsmon extracted growth factors from strictly inspected maternal placenta (Figure 29), and makes it into an injectable for intravenous or intramuscular applications, hoping to repair the function of damaged liver and combat the aging phenomenon of the whole body.

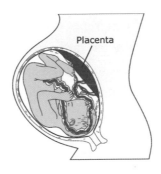

https://en.wikipedia.org/wiki/Placenta#/media/File:Placenta.svg

Figure 29. Japan used extracts of maternal placenta in 1970 to reverse aging or impaired liver function. (Image source: https://www.labiotech.eu/medical/pluristcm-cell-therapy-phase-iii/)

These two Japanese placenta companies continued to supply placenta extracts to anti-aging customers in Japan and neighboring countries in East Asia for the past 50 years. Japanese anti-aging doctors have also developed a medical tourism business model, allowing customers from all over Asia to fly to Japan every few months, receive placental injections in their clinics, and then travel around Japan.

Although placenta extract is, and probably the only, popular medicinal anti-aging product, it lacks clinical evidence. There are only a few articles published in Japanese liver journals, mostly studying its effectiveness in improving the liver function of patients with hepatitis B and C. There are no publications or case reports about the effect of placenta extract on systemic anti-aging.

In recent years, due to the aging of the population, various anti-aging methods have attracted attention of both the public, business owners, and investors alike. In Australia and New Zealand, where the animal husbandry industry is well developed, are no exception. Local health food factories (such as Alpha Laboratory) saw the successful cases of Japanese placenta companies, thought of using local pregnant deer to produce extracts of deer placenta and market it as an anti-aging supplement.

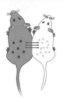

Originally, these deer placenta in New Zealand and Australia were sold through health food stores and only had limited success. Several years later, a MLM (i.e., multi-level marketing) company in southeast Asia saw the opportunity and potential of these placenta extract. They went ahead to repackage this product for the regional market. Their story attracted other supplement companies to follow in their footsteps.

Although the business of New Zealand's deer placenta lozenges has been very successful, to the best of our knowledge there is no scientific laboratory evidence nor publications that could document its efficacy. Because late entry practitioners of MLM want to expand and occupy their own market, they cannot help to exaggerate the effects of the product and to package deer placenta as an elixir for treatment of all intractable diseases. This created many customer disputes and negative reports in the media, and casts a lingering shadow on the image of the anti-aging health supplement industry.

In short, although the actual effects of the Japanese placenta injections and New Zealand deer lozenges are unknown, these are safe and legible products with more than 50 years of history. If relevant parties in the industry could have begun some basic research and conduct clinical trials to document their clinical effect, with the help of proper marketing messages to educate the public, would create a unicorn in the anti-aging industry.

10. How Did Heterochronic Parabiosis Get Back To The Centerstage Of Anti-Aging Research?

Due to political reasons, after his death, Dr. Carrel's Heterochronic Parabiosis experiment fell out of favor with mainstream scientists and physicians both in Europe and the United States. It was not until 2005 when global aging and its related degenerative diseases began to capture the attention of the medical community, which allowed the return of heterochronic parabiosis to the center stage of aging research.

A team of regenerative medical scientists led by Professor Tomas Rando of Stanford University re-examined the Heterochronic Parabiosis technology with modern experimental tools and began to look into the possibility of clinical translation of this technique which was developed by Carrel 100 years ago. (Figure 30) (Figure 31) The primary goal of Professor Rando's team was to use the Heterochronic Parabiosis experiment to explore the evidence and mechanism of how muscle tissue regenerates itself. They also hope to examine whether Heterochronic Parabiosis can affect the regeneration of other organs.

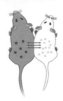

By using the young and old conjoined experiment, Rando's team not only successfully found evidence of muscle regeneration, but also confirmed its mechanism. Surprisingly, they also found that the brain and liver tissue of the older animals in the experimental old-young pair also became younger as compared to that of the old-old pair.

nature

Q   ⊗

Explore ∨   Journal info ∨   **Subscribe**

nature > letters > article

Published: 17 February 2005

Rejuvenation of aged progenitor cells by exposure to a young systemic environment

Irina M. Conboy, Michael J. Conboy, Amy J. Wagers, Eric R. Girma, Irving L. Weissman & Thomas A. Rando ✉

Nature **433**, 760–764(2005)

Figure 30. In 2005, a team of scientists, led by Professor Thomas Rando in Stanford University, specializing in regeneration of muscle tissue, started to look into potential application of Heterochronic Parabiosis in the field of anti-aging and rejuvenation medicine. (Source: nature.com)

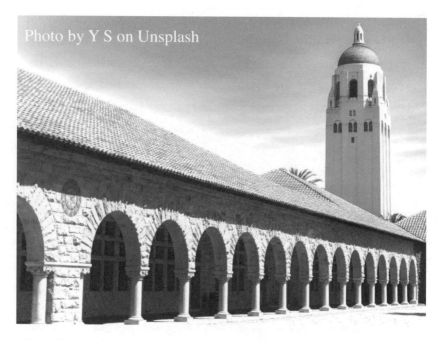

Figure 31. Stanford University, Stanford, California, USA.

Professor Rando's research initiated modern heterochronic parabiosis research with modern molecular biological techniques. Before Rando's work, there were no significant progresses in anti-aging medicine other than the well-known but decade old calorie restriction and resveratrol supplement. Rando's work had opened a new chapter in the field of modern anti-aging medicine.

Thanks to the work of Professor Rando's team and the government's focus on population aging from all developed countries, modern research on Heterochronic Parabiosis based on molecular biology has flourished since 2005. Most of the researchers use Heterochronic Parabiosis as an animal model to observe the aging process of various organs, to explore the process and mechanism of aging, and to identify targets for aging reversal drugs. It has been proved that the use of Heterochronic Parabiosis can effectively reverse aging of many internal organs, including: neurons of the brain, peripheral nerves, bones, pancreatic islet cells, liver, and skeletal muscle.

As the pathways of molecular biology involved were gradually revealed, the molecular mechanism produced by Heterochronic Parabiosis has become more and more clear. Based on these experimental works, physicians also began to organize clinical trials based on the Principal of Heterochronic Parabiosis for the treatment of various degenerative diseases. Since humans cannot be connected ethically, it has become a challenge to doctors and scientists to develop technologies to simulate the effects of Heterochronic Parabiosis observed in the old animal of the old-young pairing on the human body.

The most intuitive way to perform Heterochronic Parabiosis in a clinical setting is to replace the conjoined surgery by transfusion of young blood. This procedure seems simple, but the supply of young blood is limited, and blood transfusion has the inherited risk of rejection and infection, so it cannot be popularized.

Accordingly, Dr. Amy Wagers, a member of Professor Rando's team at Stanford, who was working in Harvard Medical School decided to analyze and compare the components in the blood of young and old mice, hoping to identify the substances that is responsible for the aging reversal, and to develop new drugs, which will solve the problems of insufficient blood supply and eliminate the risks of rejection and infection in transfusion of young blood.

11. Where Are The Aging Reversal Factors In The Blood?

The blood of humans and mice is composed of two parts: blood cells and plasma, which is composed of clotting factors and serum.

If the blood is taken out of the human body and allowed to stand still, within half an hour, the blood will automatically be separated into two parts, the clear upper serum and the lower coagulated blood cells. Plasma contains substances without life: water, electrolytes, and proteins; blood cells contain living substances, such as red blood cells, white blood cells, platelets, and trace amounts of hematopoietic stem cells and mesenchymal stem cells. (Figure 32)

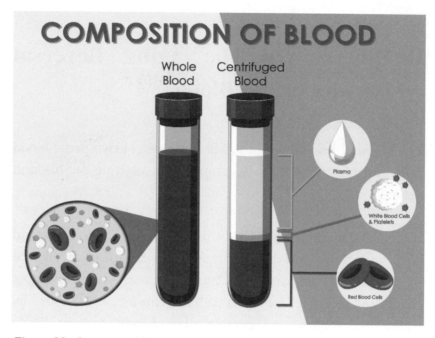

Figure 32. Contents of blood The blood can be divided into two parts, I.e., plasma and blood cells, after standing still for half an hour. Plasma contains substances without life, including water, electrolytes and proteins; blood cells contain living substances, such as red blood cells, white blood cells, platelets and a small amount of stem cells.

The life span of red blood cells is 120 days and the life spans of white blood cells and platelets is only 7 days. In addition, blood cells obviously have no direct relationship with tissue repair, it is not likely that these blood cells are the reason that aging can be reversed quickly and drastically by the young blood.

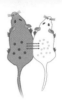

Elevian

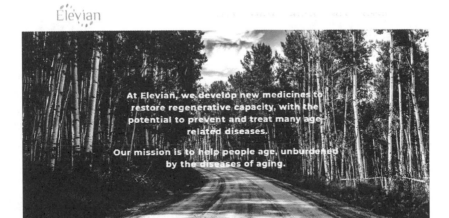

At Elevian, we develop new medicines to restore regenerative capacity, with the potential to prevent and treat many age-related diseases.

Our mission is to help people age, unburdened by the diseases of aging.

Figure 34. The Elevian Company. The GDF-11 protein was identified from the blood and injected into the mice with heart failure. As a result, it was found that the heart function can be immediately improved. Source: elevian.com

12. Who Is The Successor Of Dr. Carrel ?

The first time Dr. Carrel performed a Heterochronic Parabiosis experiment to reverse aging was around 1905. One hundred years later, in 2005, the laboratory of Professor Rando at Stanford University re-applied it and combined it with molecular biology to analyze the underlying mechanism. The technique was repeated and the work of Dr. Carrel, using conjoined surgery with a young animal to reverse aging processes of an old animal, was confirmed.

However, both in the University of Chicago and Rockefeller University, where Carrel performed his experiments, no one continued on his work until 2012.

In order to expand the scope of its influence, the Booth Business School of the University of Chicago decided to hold the first global alumni entrepreneurship competition in the newly established University of Chicago Beijing Center in the summer of 2012. The event inadvertently promoted the resurrection of Heterochronic Parabiosis research in the University of Chicago.

Although it was a small-scale competition with only 60 to 70 participants, the competition was quite fierce. To the surprise of all, the winner of the competition was a Taiwanese-American

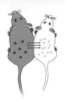

Surgeon, Fushih Pan, MD '89, PhD'86, who had never studied business before. Dr. Pan won the competition with a bottle of biological skin care products made from secretions isolated from the culture of animal mesenchymal stem cells. (Figure 35)

Certificate of Recognition

This certificate is awarded to

LOTUS BIOCHEMICAL

In recognition of outstanding achievement as a

First Place

Winner in the
Global Launchpad: Beijing
Fast-Pitch Competition
July 14, 2012

Robert Gertner
Deputy Dean and Joel F. Gemunder Professor of Strategy & Finance
The University of Chicago Booth School of Business

Waverly Deutsch
Clinical Professor of Entrepreneurship
The University of Chicago Booth School of Business

CHICAGO BOOTH | **Polsky Center**
for Entrepreneurship

Figure 35. The first place in the first Global Alumni Entrepreneurship Competition of the University of Chicago Business School in 2012 was awarded to Fushih Pan, MD,'89, PhD'86, a Taiwanese-American Plastic Surgeon who received his residency training also in the University of Chicago Hospitals.

13. Who Is Dr. Pan?

Dr. Pan (Figure 36) was born in Taipei, Taiwan. His father is a doctor of medicine and doctor of microbiology from the Imperial Kyoto University, Japan, who is a professor at the National Taiwan University School of Medicine and was the vice chairman of the World Society of Genetic Medicine during the 1998 season.

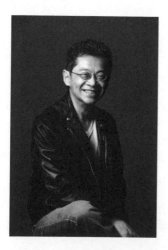

Dr. FuShih Pan

- Doctor of Medicine and Chemistry, University of Chicago, USA
- American Scientist Physician
- American Craniofacial Plastic Surgeon

Figure 36. Dr. Fushih Pan, MD, Ph.D., both from the University of Chicago, began to work on the translation of Dr. Carrel's Heterochronic Parabiosis experiment into clinical medicine in 2012.

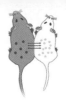

Dr. Pan graduated from the Department of Chemistry of National Taiwan University with the first place in class, he received a full scholarship from the Department of Chemistry of the University of Chicago, to continue his Ph.D. degree in Chemistry under the guidance of Professor Takeshi Oka, Diplomate of the American Academy of Sciences. His thesis was using high resolution infrared laser spectroscopy to study chemical reactions of molecular ions occurring in gaseous plasma. These are of fundamental importance for understanding the chemistry that occurs in the molecular clouds in outer space.

At that time, Professor Yang Nian-zu, an organic chemist, was responsible for the Pre-Med program at the College of The University of Chicago. When he learned about this MSTP program, he strongly recommended Dr. Pan, at that time a Ph.D. candidate, to the Dean Joseph Ceithamal of the Medical School. The two teamed up with Professor Liao Shuz-hong of the Ben May Cancer Research Center of the University of Chicago Hospitals to overcome all difficulties and make Dr. Pan the only student who did not have a US citizenship or permanent residency to study in this prestige MSTP program.

After completing his medical degree, Dr. Pan continued his training in the combined plastic and reconstructive surgery residency program in The University of Chicago Hospitals. While he was a resident, Dr. Pan worked with Professor Chin-Tu Chen from the Department of Medical Physics at School of

Medicine of the University of Chicago to developed a technology to detect the degree of hypoxia in the yeast cells by the fluorescence generated by NADH (Reduction state of Nicotinamide Adenine Dinucleotide) molecule after shined by a 337nm nitrogen pulse laser.

He also participated in the cutting-edge regenerative medicine research of Professor Raphael C. Lee of Massachusetts Institute of Technology before and continued after he was relocated to the University of Chicago on the use of co-polymers to rescue muscle cells injuries by electric burns.

In 1994, Dr. Pan left the University of Chicago to study cranio-facial surgery at the Children's Hospital Of Philadelphia under Dr. Linton Whitaker and Dr. Scott Bartlet as the number one draft in the global match. At the same time, he also served as a lecturer in plastic surgery at the School of Medicine at the University of Pennsylvania of the ivy league.

With a background in physics and chemistry, Dr. Pan utilized the newly developed 3D scanning technology to explore the short term and long-term result of the craniofacial surgery. For which, he was awarded the basic research award of Ivy Society of Plastic Surgery.

At this time, the School of Medicine of the University of Pennsylvania began to pay attention to the importance of

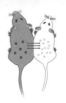

regenerative medicine in the wake of population aging. Professor Linton A. Whitaker, then the chair of the Department of Plastic Surgery, instructed Dr. Pan to research the relationship between regenerative medicine and anti-aging medicine. Dr. Pan subsequently conducted a series of experiments to explore the basic theories of regenerative processes in craniofacial surgery and published several important research papers. One of the papers confirmed the importance of scaffold materials for skull regeneration, and the other paper measured the tension required for skull regeneration, because these works are an inspiration for the development of regenerative medicine in the future, he was awarded the 1994 Basic Science Research Award of the American Maxillofacial Surgery Society.

Dr. Pan originally planned to return to his alma mater at the University of Chicago, to continue his work on craniofacial surgery. At that time, he had the chance to meet with Dr. Zhang Zhao-xiong from Chang Gung Memorial Hospital, who at the request of Taiwan's Vice President Lien Chan (PhD' Department of Political Science, the University of Chicago and Director of the Board of Trustees, The University of Chicago) was visiting United States to recruit talents in the field of biomedical research to return to Taiwan. During the brief session, Dr. Pan thought that this might be the last chance for return to his hometown, decided to return his offers from several of the American Universities and returned to Taipei, Taiwan in the summer of 1995.

Dr. Pan found that the craniofacial surgery market in Taiwan was dominated by Chang Gung Memorial Hospital led by Dr. Samuel Nordoff, as a result, decided to apply his knowledge and skill in craniofacial surgery to establish a private clinic focused on facial reconstructive and cosmetic surgeries. In the next five years, he completed nearly two thousand facelifts and became the leading endoscopy and facelift surgeons in Taiwan at that time.

Through the recommendation of Dr. Zhao Xia-fu, a famous gastroenterologist and seasoned investor in Taiwan, Mr. Zhang Zhong-pu, the Chairman of the China Development Company owned by the Kuo Ming Tang Party,invited Dr. Pan to serve as the superintendent of their newly acquired China County Hospital at the millennium to transformed it into the first hospital focused in consumer medicine and surgeries in Asia.

In order to help more people with what he has learned in the field of chemistry and medicine, Dr. Pan decided to leave the administrative and management post at the expiration of his term of office to begin his task to create an anti-aging technology company as a medical scientist.

At this time, Dr. Marc Hedrick of the University of California, Los Angeles successfully isolated mesenchymal stem cells of the adipose tissue (i.e. ADSC, Adipose Derived Stem Cells) obtained from the lipoaspirate of the common liposuction procedure. This

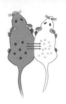

Lotus Biochemical Company was the first company to use a mass spectrometer to analyze the chemical components in natural products and conditioned media obtained from the stem cell cultures under various conditions, hoping to design formulas for anti-aging supplements. In order to respond to the trend of non-invasive treatments in the plastic surgery market, Dr. Pan also used these stem cell conditioned media to develop several topicals for skin rejuvenation and hair follicle regeneration, for which he was awarded the first position of the first global alumni entrepreneurship in the Booth School of Business at the University of Chicago.

14. How Did Dr. Pan Returned To The Clan?

When participating in the business school entrepreneurship competition at the University of Chicago Center in Beijing, Dr. Pan also visited the Display Wall of University of Chicago Nobel Prize winners. (Figure 37) Dr. Pan first visited the photo of two Chinese Nobel Prize winners in Physics, Dr. Yang Zhen-ning and Dr. Li Zheng-dao. At this time, Dr. Pan was attracted by the photo of another Nobel Prize winner located at the right upper corner. He took a closer look. It was Dr. Alexis Carrel, whom he had never paid any attention to during his more than ten years at the University of Chicago Medical School and University of Chicago Hospitals. (Figure 38)

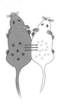

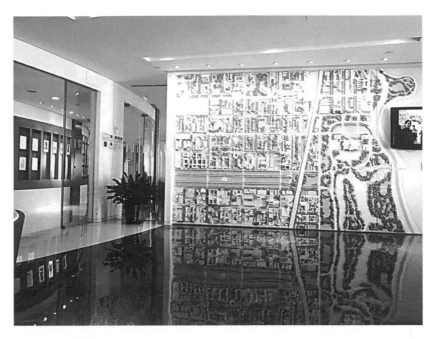

Figure 37. The Nobel Prize display wall located at the University of Chicago Beijing Center.

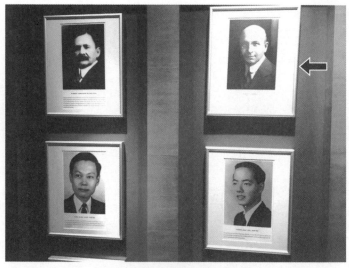

Figure 38. The portrait of Dr. Alexis Carrel is hung on the Nobel Prize display wall next to that of the two Chinese's Nobel Prize winner of Physics in 1957 at the Nobel Wall in the University of Chicago Beijing Center

Out of curiosity, Dr. Pan immediately searched the background of Dr. Carrel through Baidu and learned about the incredible work of Dr. Carrel and his political controversies. At that time, Dr. Pan suddenly recalled that: while he was developing the skin and hair follicle products using conditioned media collected from cultures of adipose derived stem cells, a research assistant came to tell him: "the hair of old mouse grows after 3 months of topical application; at the same time, the old and bald animal also become lively and active, just like a young mouse". (Figure 39) Dr. Pan thought: just like topical medications could be absorbed through the skin and hair follicles to enter the circulatory system

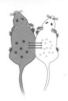

of the body, this phenomenon is actually the systemic effect of secretions of stem cells absorbed by the skin of mice. Although the rate absorption of conditioned media through the mouse skin is unknown, however, after long-term application, the concentration of secretions in the body might have had gradually increased to enabled similar rejuvenation effects like what was observed in the old-young conjoined experiments performed by Dr. Carrel 106 years ago in the Surgery Department of the University of Chicago."

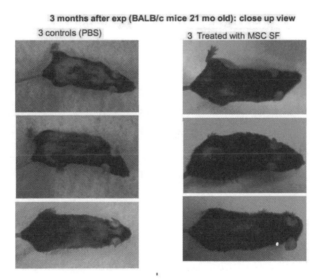

Figure 39. Experiment of smearing stem cell secretions on the skin of old mice. During the product testing phase of the development of stem cell skin care products, the research assistant discovered that after the old mice had grown new hairs, they also became lively and active, just like young mice.

Because the effect of this hypothetical type of Heterochronic Parabiosis is achieved through skin absorption, Dr. Pan decided to named it as Transdermal Heterochronic Parabiosis (Trans: Pass, Dermo: Skin, Heterochronic: different age, Parabiosis: living together) and immediately add this to the title of his PowerPoint for the final competition, to deliver a powerful message to shock all the judges.

Dr. Pan, who proposed the theory of transdermal Heterochronic Parabiosis, wants to apply it for the anti-aging of the entire body. Because human skin is tighter than the mouse skin, which forbids any molecule with a molecular weight greater than 500 Daltons to penetrate. Although stem cell topicals do have a good clinical result in rejuvenation of the skin and hair follicles, however, based on the Franz test performed by Dr. Pan's laboratory almost none can penetrate the human skin. As a result, there still were no systemic anti-aging effects observed among hundreds of users of the skin and hair topicals made of conditioned media of stem cells. Better introduction methods needed to be developed before further attempts for achieving systemic anti-aging effects should be initiated.

Dr. Pan had attempted to increase the absorption by heat, ultrasonic delivering devices, and micro-roller, however, none were effective to result in any signs and symptoms that indicated systemic rejuvenation. Dr. Pan had also considered delivering the stem cell solutions with a skin-tight mask made by the dental acting method just like what he used for his research of craniofacial surgery back in 1994 at the Children's Hospital of Philadelphia. However, the process was too long and uncomfortable, which is unacceptable for cosmetic clients and could not even be attempted.

On 4/5/2014, it was the traditional tomb sweeping day, i.e., Qing-ming Festival, in Taiwan. The junior brother of Dr. Pan, Pan Fu-tao was driving the family to pay their respect to the late Prof. Pan I-hung within the Yanming mountain in suburban Taipei. Pan Fu-tao mentioned to Dr. Pan, that the patent for 3D printing expired a few months ago, and the printing cost was greatly reduced. Since Dr. Pan has had clinical experience in 3D applications back in the era at the University of Pennsylvania and had been seeking methods to increase absorption of stem cell secretions, Dr. Pan began to evaluate the possibility of create a personalized facial device that can accelerate transcutaneous absorption of stem cell secretions.

The mask was designed not only for increased absorption of the large molecules throughout the skin, but also function as the retention or molding device of the face. The 3D anti-aging mask entered the market in the Fall of 2014 (Figure 40), and was awarded two US design patents (Figure 41) (Figure 42). Clinical studies have shown that wearing a 3D anti-aging mask can effectively stop the sagging of the face in particular to the jowl region and rejuvenates the skin at the same time (Figure 43).

Although the personalized 3D mask greatly increased the absorption of the stem cell secretions and resulted in great results of facial rejuvenation, however, the introduction of 3D masks still failed to bring up any systemic anti-aging effect.

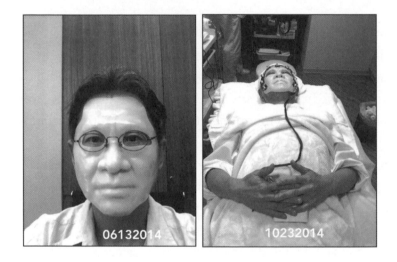

Figure 40. The 3D anti-aging mask was created in 2014. Dr. Pan was the first user.

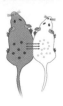

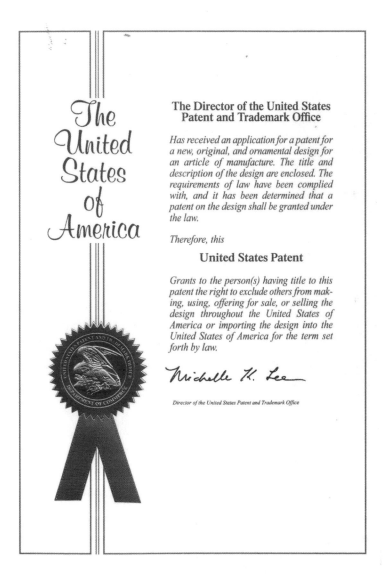

The Director of the United States
Patent and Trademark Office

Has received an application for a patent for a new, original, and ornamental design for an article of manufacture. The title and description of the design are enclosed. The requirements of law have been complied with, and it has been determined that a patent on the design shall be granted under the law.

Therefore, this

United States Patent

Grants to the person(s) having title to this patent the right to exclude others from making, using, offering for sale, or selling the design throughout the United States of America or importing the design into the United States of America for the term set forth by law.

Director of the United States Patent and Trademark Office

Figure 41. The 3D anti-aging mask was awarded two US patents.

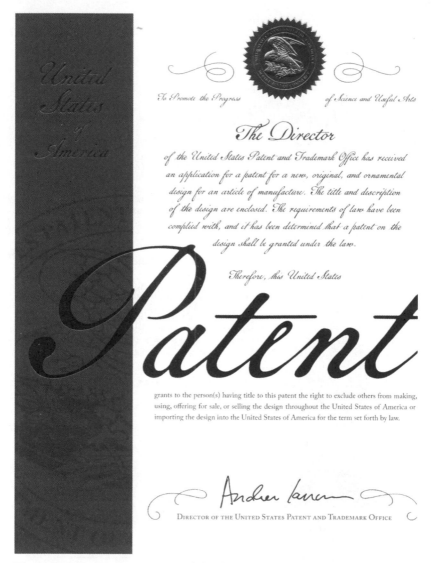

To Promote the Progress *of Science and Useful Arts*

The Director

of the United States Patent and Trademark Office has received
an application for a patent for a new, original, and ornamental
design for an article of manufacture. The title and description
of the design are enclosed. The requirements of law have been
complied with, and it has been determined that a patent on the
design shall be granted under the law.

Therefore, this United States

Patent

grants to the person(s) having title to this patent the right to exclude others from making,
using, offering for sale, or selling the design throughout the United States of America or
importing the design into the United States of America for the term set forth by law.

DIRECTOR OF THE UNITED STATES PATENT AND TRADEMARK OFFICE

Figure 42. The 3D anti-aging mask has been awarded two US patents.

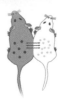

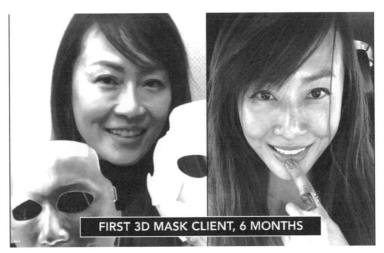

FIRST 3D MASK CLIENT, 6 MONTHS

Figure 43. Clinical study found that wearing a 3D anti-aging mask can effectively stop the sagging of the customer's face and rejuvenate the skin.

Among 2,000 customers who wear the masks on a regular basis (i.e., three or four times a week for 30 minutes each) for three months, less than 20% reported systemic anti-aging effects like: feeling more energetic, experiencing improvements in sleep quality, etc…

Because stem cell transplantation is limited by the first pass (i.e., filtering effect of the capillary of the lungs), stem cell activation is limited by the supply and limited dosing, transdermal delivery of stem cell secretion is limited by the efficiency of absorption through the human skin, it is impossible to produce systemic anti-aging effects clinically.

To the best of our knowledge, almost all of the systemic anti-aging attempts are only limited to successes in animal experiments. The dream of mankind to reverse aging for the entire body is still far away.

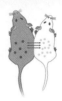

15. Can The Effect Of Heterochronic Parabiosis Happened For A Different Reason ?

Although the Heterochronic Parabiosis experiment has shown amazing effects in animal experiments, its clinical application has been stagnant. Until very recently, there has been a lack of reliable clinical trials since Dr. Carrel's observations in 1906. In order to resolve this puzzle, scientists and physicians alike are forced to re-examine how Heterochronic Parabiosis reverses aging and hope to establish new anti-aging methods based on better understanding of the underlying mechanism for Heterochronic Parabiosis.

After conjoined experiments of one old and one young mouse, they will establish collateral circulations which allows them to share what is inside of their blood and functions of their internal organs exert on the blood. The effects of internal organs were ruled out by Dr. Carrel and other early scientists by removing them one by one, as the result, the anti-aging effect of Heterochronic Parabiosis should definitely be resulted from the sharing of blood.

Since the blood is a liquid, the old and young blood can easily be mixed; half of the young blood will enter the body of the old animal, and half of the blood in the old animal will enter the body of the young animal. Likewise, the concentration of various beneficial or harmful substances in the blood will also decrease or increase by 50% respectively.

What's interesting is that because only old animals become younger has clinical and economic value (in other words, making younger animals older has no clinical benefit or economical value), for the past century almost all of the scientists and physicians who studied Heterochronic Parabiosis have focused on how to make old animals younger, there were no one had studied how to use Heterochronic Parabiosis conjoined surgery to make young animals grow old.

One of the members of Professor Rando's 2005 research team is Dr. Irina Conboy from Russia. In the 1990s, she was studying autoimmunity with Dr. Patricia Jones at Stanford University. After married to Dr. Michael Conboy, the couple collaborated to become a well-known husband and wife stem cell anti-aging research team in the Bay Area.

When Dr. Irina Conboy was doing postdoctoral research in Professor Rando's laboratory, her main research topic was to understand how aging inhibits the ability of muscle cells to regenerate. When she was collaborating with Irv Weissman, she

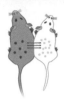

come across the conjoined Heterochronic Parabiosis experiments.

In 2008, Dr. Conboy left Stanford University to the neighboring University of California at Berkeley to continue her works in using conjoined old-young animal experiments to study various aspects of aging.

In order to understand the mystery of the ineffectiveness of transfusion of young blood in the clinic setting, she deviated from the traditional framework and examined the results of the Heterochronic Parabiosis experiment from a different angle. She thought : just like the blood of young animals may contain factors which are beneficial to the aging animals; the blood of aging animals might also contain substances that can accelerate the aging of the organs of young animals.

The blind spot she saw that no one had previously noticed was "aging blood may contain substances that inhibit organ function". She went ahead to conduct a simple experiment to prove her hypothesis. She designed an intermittent Heterochronic Parabiosis experiment, where she injected certain amount of young blood into the aging animals, and injected same amount of blood from the old animal into the young animal repeatedly at a certain interval. She observed that the suppression power of the aging blood on the function of the youthful organ of a young animal greatly exceeds the beneficial effects of blood from the young animal to the aging organs of the old animal (Figure 44)!

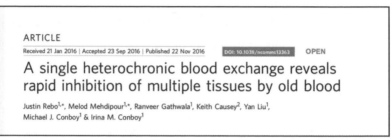

ARTICLE

Received 21 Jan 2016 | Accepted 23 Sep 2016 | Published 22 Nov 2016   DOI: 10.1038/ncomms13363   OPEN

A single heterochronic blood exchange reveals rapid inhibition of multiple tissues by old blood

Justin Rebo[1,*], Melod Mehdipour[1,*], Ranveer Gathwala[1], Keith Causey[2], Yan Liu[1], Michael J. Conboy[1] & Irina M. Conboy[1]

THE HARMFUL EFFETS OF OLD PLASMA IS GREATER THAN THE BENEFICIAL EFFECTS OF YOUNG PLASMA.

Figure 44. The blood of aging animals was injected into the body of young animals and vice versa. It was found that the extent of aging blood inhibited the function of young organs was far greater than the beneficial effect of the young blood on the function of aging organs. Source: nature.com

To put it simply, in addition to the beneficial substances in young blood, aging blood also contains harmful substances; and the influence of harmful substances is far greater than the beneficial substances; this is the origin of the important concept of "old blood is poisonous".

This phenomenon can be explained using the model of automobile transmission. Just like a car has an accelerator pedal and a brake pedal; aging blood is like a brake to organs, and the young blood is like an accelerator to organ.

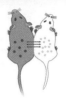

If there is a lot of aging blood in the body, it is like you are stepping on the brakes hard, no matter how you step on the accelerator, that is, transplanting a lot of stem cells or adding a lot of growth hormones and cytokines, the function of the organs will not be improved. If a small amount of aging substances can be removed, it is like relaxing a little brake force. Then, if you step on the accelerator harder, the car will start to move forward, which means that the organ function can be improved.

If the brakes can be completely released, that is, the harmful substances in the aging blood can be completely eliminated, then the car will run forward if you just lightly step on the gas paddle, which means that by adding a little beneficial substance, the organ function will be improved quickly.

This major discovery that old blood is toxic not only explains why the Heterochronic Parabiosis conjoined experiment cannot be simulated in a clinical setting by simply transfusing blood from young people, but also opens a pathway in making the Heterochronic Parabiosis experiment clinically feasible!

16. What Should Be The Anti-Aging Treatment Be Re-Designed Based on The Current Understandings Of Heterochronic Parabiosis?

With the new understanding that old blood is poisonous, scientists from various countries engaged in Heterochronic Parabiosis have redesigned their research directions and experimental methods accordingly, each showing their strengths, and studying how to improve the function of aging organs. In Stanford University, Professor Rando's team mainly focuses on muscle regeneration while Professor Wyss-Coray's team focuses on the regeneration of neurons of the brain and documenting proteomics at different ages. Dr. Wagers' team in Harvard focuses on identifying effective substance in the young blood that can improve the function of the heart, while Dr. Conboys' (husband and wife) team in University of California, Berkley focused on identifying and measuring the effect of harmful proteins in the old blood on the function of various organs.

Since most of the researchers are scientists rather than physicians, the research direction is still heavily weighted towards the study of the molecular biology of Heterochronic Parabiosis.

On the clinical side, the main promoters are only Dr. Dobri Kiprov and Dr. Pan. Dr. Kiprov advocated using the existing plasma exchange machine (Plasmapheresis Machine) to eliminate toxic substances, and using the existing pharmatheutical products like serum albumin and immunoglobulin as the plasma replacements.

Dr. Pan generally agrees with Dr. Kiprov's approach. He also believes that an accurate anti-aging model is key to the design of new anti-aging programs. The previously anti-aging model was modified and the effect of the toxic factor of old blood was added (Figure 45). The correct model should be used to explain why the stem cell transplantation and stem cell activation methods in the past failed to reverse the causes of aging before it is used to design new clinical programs.

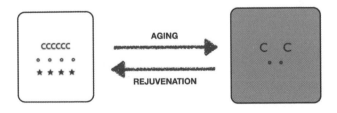

Figure 45. New aging model. It explains why stem cell transplantation and stem cell activation failed to reverse aging in the past.

Dr. Pan used the new model to re-examine stem cell transplantation and explained why the procedure cannot produce significant systemic anti-aging effects. In addition to the problem of lung filtration; the stem cells used in clinical settings are usually cultured in a clean laboratory environment before the implantation procedure. As a result, when it enters the stream of toxin-containing old blood of the vein, the survival rate becomes very low. (Figure 46)

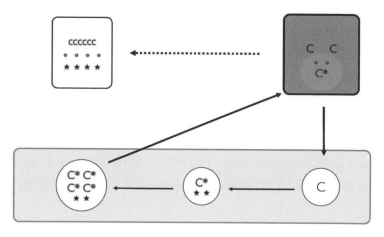

Figure 46. Transplanted stem cells are cultured in the clean laboratory environment before being implanted into the human body. After entering the human body from the vein, the toxins in the old blood could kill most of the implanted stem cells.

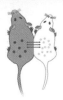

Some physicians believe that if the customers who have received detoxification before implantation of stem cells can get better results, however, even the survival rates of stem cell can be improved, there are still short of activation signaling factors; the implanted stem cells will quickly enter a dormant state and could not perform any repair function. (Figure 47)

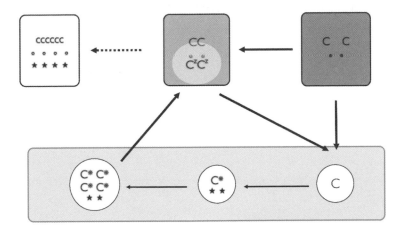

Figure 47. If you go through detoxification before implanting the stem cells, the survival rate of stem cells can be improved, but the lack of activation factors still prohibit them from beginning their repair functions.

With the help of his background in physical chemistry, Dr. Pan repeatedly evaluated the modified anti-aging model, finally succeeded in redesigning an effective anti-aging program based on the Principle of Heterochronic Parabiosis.

117

He broke down the effect of Heterochronic Parabiosis experiment into three parts (Figure 48), the first step (A) is to eliminate harmful substances in the old plasma, the second step (B) is to supplement the detoxified plasma with beneficial substances, and the third and last step (C) is to transplant adequate number of stem cells based on the measurement of the number of stem cells in the plasma. Finally, the three steps must be performed in order, otherwise the effect of conjoined Heterochronic Parabiosis cannot be fully simulated.

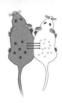

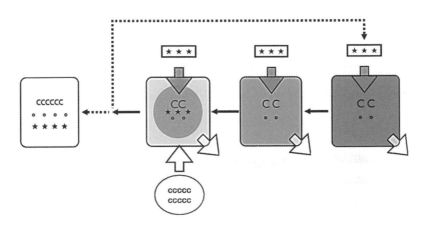

Figure 48. Three key steps of newly designed anti-aging therapy based on the Principle of Heterochronic Parabiosis. The Heterochronic Parabiosis therapy proposed by Dr. Pan contains three parts: eliminate harmful substances, supplement beneficial factors, and transplant small amounts of stem cells. All of which are indispensable.

The human body could be regarded as an aquarium. It is usually equipped with simple ventilation and filtering devices to perform water quality maintenance work. However, if the water were never changed, there will be residual protein molecules in the water, which will gradually form harmful protein aggregates. The fish schools would not be healthy.

If you want to increase the number of healthy fish in the fish tank, you must first remove part of the contaminated water, followed by addition of some clean water and nutrients before transferring healthy new fish into the tank. This concept of "fishing must first raise water" (Figure 49) is very similar to the concept of "health must first nourish blood (clearing)" embedded in the clinical Heterochronic Parabiosis program designed by Dr. Pan.

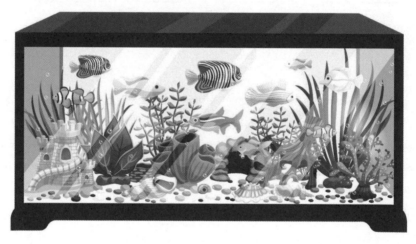

Figure 49. To raise fish, you must raise the water first. The concept of "health must first nourish blood" developed over the past 100 years is the same as the concept of "fish must first nourish water".

17. How To Detoxify Aging Plasma?

There are three steps in Heterochronic Parabiosis (anti-aging) therapy. The first step is to reduce the substances that are harmful to the stem cells in the aging blood. The second step is to increase the substances that are beneficial to stem cells in the young blood. The third is to transplant a small amount of stem cells into the plasma if there is shortage of them (mostly for clients or patients who are more than 80 years old. (Figure 50)

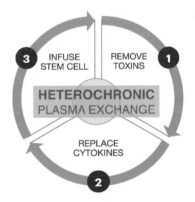

Figure 50. The three steps of Heterochronic Parabiosis therapy. The first step of Heterochronic Parabiosis therapy is to reduce the substances that are harmful to stem cells in the aging blood, the second step is to increase the substances that are beneficial to stem cells in the young blood, and the last step is to import young and healthy stem cells with regulatory functions.

The first step which is also the key step for the process of Heterochronic Parabiosis is to reduce substances that are harmful to the stem cells in aging blood.

Although the importance of blood toxins for aging was not proven until Dr. Irina Conboy's work in 2016, the concept of detoxification is not a new one and very common in traditional medicine.

The detoxification mechanism in the human body includes three parts. (Figure 51) The first part is to reduce the number of toxic substances that enter the human body. The second part is to increase the efficiency of the human liver to decompose the harmful substances. The third part is to accelerate the excretion of residual substances produced by the liver.

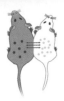

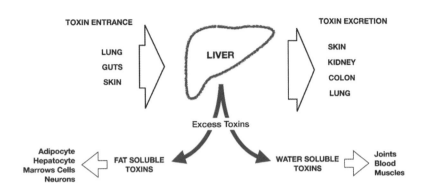

Figure 51. The metabolic process of toxic substances in humans. Toxins are absorbed through the breath (lungs), skin (pores) and diet (intestinal tract). After entering the body, they are transported to the liver by the bloodstream to be decomposed. The residual of decomposed toxins are excreted through the skin, urine, defecation and breathing. Toxins that cannot be metabolized are stored in various organs and blood.

Image source: http://www.santannaturalmedicine.com/2015/03/03/spring-cleaning-a-guide-to-detoxification/

Most of the toxic substances in the human body enter the human body through the lungs, skin or digestive system; the substances that enter the human body from the lungs are substances related to air pollution, including: PM2.5 particles or toxic gases such as sulfur dioxide; those that enter the human body from the skin are harmful substances like: free radicals generated by the ultraviolet radiations in the sunlight, accidentally contacted chemicals, cosmetics or skin care products that are poor-quality. Heavy metals, plastics, and food processing additives, might also enter our body by absorption from the stomach and intestines.

When these harmful substances enter the human body, they will gradually find their way into the capillaries, and then be taken to the liver, which specializes in processing toxic substances, by blood circulation. There are various enzymes in the liver that can catabolize these toxic substances into smaller chemical molecules which might be excreted by the kidneys, skin, large intestine, and lungs.

Under normal circumstances, toxic substances can be completely eliminated after entering the human body by the liver. However, with the increase in age, change in living habits might gradually increase the number of toxic substances entering the body, at the same time the detoxification capacity of the liver, kidneys, large intestine, lungs and skin reduced, which resulted in the accumulation of toxic substances and begin to inhibit normal function of various organs.

Toxic substances can be divided into two categories. The first category is toxic substances that are easily dissolved in fat, such as pesticides, pesticide residues, hormones, etc. These substances are also easier to deposit in fat cells, bone marrow cells, liver, as well as the central nervous system.

The second category of toxic substances are water-soluble, such as nicotine, toxic gases, and other chemical substances. Water-soluble toxins are easy to accumulate in joints, connective tissues, muscles, and blood.

When the accumulated toxic substances reach a threshold, it will begin to produce various side effects which will eventually result in pathological processes, e.g., allergies, arthritis, cardiovascular disease, autoimmune diseases, hormonal imbalance, skin pigmentation, obesity, and degenerative diseases of the nervous system.

Detoxification plays a very important role in maintaining health. Traditional medicine usually emphasizes the importance of detoxification, these range from massage, cupping techniques in folk therapy, to various natural or brewed enzymes that can expel gastrointestinal toxins, and so on. For toxins in the blood, there are techniques such as chelation therapy for removal of heavy metals, plasma exchange and kidney dialysis to remove toxic metabolites like ammonia. In recent years, there has also been psychotherapy that uses meditation to eliminate toxins from the central nervous system.

Since the first step in Heterochronic Parabiosis is to eliminate toxins in the blood that can inhibit the normal function of stem cells, blood detoxification methods are needed.

There are two traditional blood detoxification therapies. The first is the relatively simple chelation therapy. It uses a chemical called EDTA (Ethylene-Diamine-Tetra-Acetic Acid). This molecule has two negative charges to bind to heavy metals with two positive charges (Figure 52) to form a conjugate that might be excreted through the kidneys. Clinical studies have shown that chelation therapy can eliminate heavy metals and promote proliferation of vascular endothelial cells.

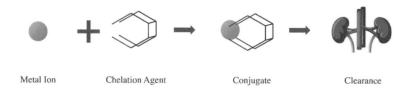

Metal Ion   Chelation Agent   Conjugate   Clearance

Figure 52. Schematic diagram of EDTA chelation therapy. Clinical studies have shown that EDTA therapy can eliminate heavy metals and can promote the proliferation of vascular endothelial cells.

Chelation agents can cause a burning sensation in the blood vessels during injection, the treatment process must be carried at a very slow speed. Moreover, at least a dozen such treatments must be completed to see any clinical effects. Since each treatment costs 350 to 700 US dollars, a course of treatment can easily surpass ten thousands USD, and is usually not reimbursed by the insurance. The acceptance of chelation therapy is therefore not very good.

The second method of blood detoxification is blood exchange (i.e., plasmapheresis), also known as blood cleansing. It requires a medical device that first draws blood out of the body; then separates the blood cells from plasma (the blood cells are partly returned to the body), followed by centrifugal or permeable membrane filtration to separate chemical substances of specific molecular weight and discard the unwanted portion out of the body. (Figure 53)

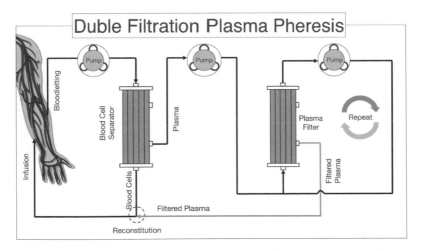

Figure 53. Schematic diagram of blood exchange. Plasmapheresis, also known as blood washing. Filter out large molecular weight substances such as cholesterol and triglycerides through centrifugation or permeable membrane filtration. The blood cells are transferred back to the body.

The third method of removing harmful substances in blood is to extract a small portion of the blood from the human body, and then remove harmful substances with various filters or inject ozone to remove free radicals in a sterile fashion before returning it to the body. Although this method of plasma detoxification is fast, it can only process 300 ml to 500 ml of blood each time, and it costs around 350-500USD. Therefore, if the blood of the whole body is to be processed, the cost will also become very high. Furthermore, since the blood is processed outside the body manually, it is impossible to avoid operator errors and the risk of infection. It is currently only practiced in mainland China.

The last method to eliminate toxins in blood is also the simplest, most effective and cheapest, this is bloodletting or phlebotomy. The blood in a person's body is roughly 7.5% of the body weight. For a 65 kg person, the total amount of blood in his body is about 5000 ml or 5 kg. Under normal circumstances, 40% of the human blood is blood cells and 60% is plasma, as the result, a 65 kg person only has 3000 ml of plasma. This is the reason why blood banks limit the amount of blood donation for a man to less than 500 ml, and for a female to less than 250 ml. By removing 150ml of plasma, 3% (150ml/3000ml) of all toxins in the human body can be eliminated completely.

This method is simple, fast and effective, and there is almost no cost. In addition to quickly and effectively eliminating all toxins in the blood, bloodletting can stimulate the vitality of

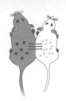

hematopoietic and mesenchymal stem cells in the bone marrow as well as reduce the concentration of iron in the blood. A recent large-scale human study in Germany shows that if too many iron atoms accumulate in the human body, life span will be reduced. This confirms that bloodletting is a safe, simple, effective and multi-purpose detoxification method.

18. Where Are The Beneficial Factors For Stem Cell In The Blood?

After excluding the harmful substance for the stem cells from the aging blood, the second step of the Heterochronic Parabiosis Therapy is to supplement the substances that are beneficial to the stem cells in the young blood.

But where are these beneficial substances for stem cells located in the blood? In order to translate Heterochronic Parabiosis into clinical practice, the source of young blood is the biggest obstacle.

In terms of animal experiments, Dr. Carrel connected the old and the young animals surgically to allow them to establish a shared microvascular circulatory system which enabled the old animal to receive blood of young animals for the purpose of reversing the function of aging organs. This method has been used in the laboratory until now.

Since people cannot be conjoined, there are only four potential sources of young blood. The first is the blood stored when you are young (autologous), the second is the blood of others (allogeneic), the third is animal blood (xenographic), and the

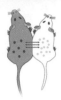

fourth and last is chemically synthesized blood (man-made or artificial blood).

Other than the blood stored in the youth, the use of other people's or animal blood will inevitably have inherited risk of rejection and infection.

Although chemical synthesis of blood has been the interest of scientists for many decades throughout the world, it is still not achieved.

Fortunately, after careful analysis, the substances in the young blood that are beneficial to the stem cell should be proteins in the plasma. In order to avoid the risk of rejection, we could separate the plasma from the blood cells using centrifugation or membrane filtration technologies. We can then apply Pasteur's sterilization method to the remaining plasma, by which most of the bacteria and viruses that cause infectious diseases can be eliminated.

In short, if Pasteurized young plasma is used to replace young blood, the risk of rejection of using young blood can be completely eliminated, and the chance of infection is also very low.

19. What Are The Potential Sources Of Young Plasma ?

1.Autologous Plasma (plasma from patient himself or herself)

Theoretically, customers can store their own blood or plasma at a young age, and then re-infuse it after 50 years of age. Since the concept of Heterochronic Parabiosis only began to gain attention after 2005, even the wealthiest who are unscrupulous in the pursuit of immortality should not have stored their own young blood or plasma. Moreover, the activity of blood or plasma will decline after many years of storage; in addition to the high cost of low temperature storage, it is not a good method.

2.Allogeneic Plasma (plasma from other people)

The blood bank should be the easiest source for plasma of another person, i.e., FFP (Fresh Frozen Plasma). However, as the 2016 study by Stanford University showed: aging blood actually contains toxins that might inhibit stem cells and organ function. Unless you can find a reliable, clean and young donor from your family, there is a risk of receiving toxins residing in other people's plasma. In other words, if you incidentally received the

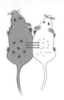

blood of an older donor or someone has poor lifestyles, it might actually accelerate the aging processes.

The law and regulations regarding blood donation varies in different countries. The age of blood donation in the United States is over 18 years old and the age can be specified. While in other countries, it may require the age of up to 18 before they could donate and cannot be specified. Since young blood transfusion is an intuitive approach to practice Heterochronic Parabiosis in a clinical setting, there are several companies that see this business opportunity to raise substantial funding to set up blood transfusion centers across the US. They recruit college students who need money to sell blood to wealthy customers who want to fight against aging by receiving young blood or plasma transfusions.

Because the blood or plasma donated by college students is type matched, there is no risk of rejection. Although the blood of college students has also been tested for common pathogens of various infectious diseases, the incubation period of viruses like AIDS and other unknown diseases can be as long as half a year, so the risk of infection could not be completely ruled out.

Of course, we can consider using adolescent plasma that is younger than that of college students, but adolescent donors are usually prohibited in most countries, the source is limited and the price is high.

As for baby or newborn plasma, it is even more difficult to obtain. In particular, the weight of a baby or newborn is only three to four kilograms, the total blood volume is only one or two hundred milliliters at most, therefore only less than 10 milliliters of blood can be collected each time. If their serum is to be used for a Heterochronic Parabiosis treatment, it will require at least a dozen young children as donors for each session, which is fundamentally a fantasy in any modern society.

3.Xenographic Plasma (plasma from the animal)

There is no supply or age issue of plasma from an animal source. If the animal's blood cells are separated by centrifugation, and the remaining plasma is processed by pasteurization, the risk of bacterial or viral infection could also be eliminated and it appears to be a good source of young plasma.

Unfortunately, animals which are similar in size with humans have a deadly infectious disease called prion disease. (Figure 54) This disease is not caused by bacteria or viruses, but by a very special protein. It can replicate and has the ability to infect, and the lethality rate is 100%!

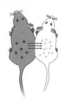

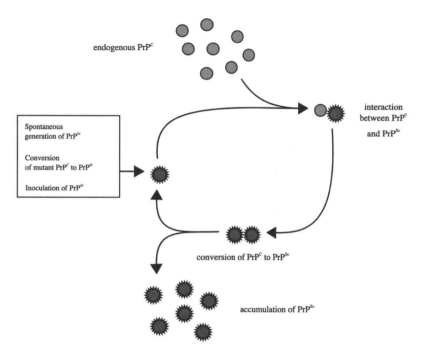

endogenous PrP^c

Spontaneous
generation of PrP^{Sc}

Conversion
of mutant PrP^c to PrP^{Sc}

Inoculation of PrP^{Sc}

interaction
between PrP^c
and PrP^{Sc}

conversion of PrP^c to PrP^{Sc}

accumulation of PrP^{Sc}

Figure 54. Animal serum may have an infectious protein called Prion. This disease is commonly known as mad cow disease in cattle. The same form of disease can occur in sheep, pigs, horses, and deer. Image source: wikiwand.com

Because currently we do not have any means to detect this pathogen, the only way to diagnose the illness is by autopsy, i.e., biopsy of the brain.

This disease is commonly known as mad cow disease. The same form of disease can occur in sheep, pigs, horses, and deer. The only way to eliminate it is high temperature disinfection, but after high temperature disinfection, the substances in the plasma that are beneficial to stem cells will also be completely destroyed and will not have any beneficial effect.

Therefore, although animal plasma seems to be a good choice, transfusion of which is prohibited by laws and regulations because of safety considerations. To the best of our knowledge, there are no establishments (hospitals, clinics, or companies) engaged in this type of practice currently.

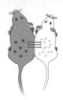

20. Why Is The Treatment Offered By Ambrosia Ineffective?

The function of aging organs in old animals can be reversed by connecting the old animal to a young animal through surgery. Since humans cannot be connected, many physicians intuitively think of transfusing young blood to simulate it in clinical practice.

There have been rumors in Asian countries for thousands of years that those in power or ascetics used young serum to keep their youth. In Europe and the United States, stories about how humans manage to obtain immortality by drawing young blood also have a history of hundreds of years. However, there are no reports in any scientific or clinical literature describing these therapies until very recently.

It was not until 2014 that Dr. Wyss-Coray of Stanford University formally proposed the concept of intermittent Heterochronic Parabiosis in animal experiments, which also brought the concept of intermittent Heterochronic Parabiosis to the attention of clinical doctors.

Among all the physicians and scientists who wish to make Heterochronic Parabiosis feasible clinically, the person with the most entrepreneurial spirit should be Dr. Jesse Karmazin. He is a graduate of Stanford University School of Medicine. When he was in medical school, he heard about experiments related to Heterochronic Parabiosis, and intuitively felt that this was an excellent business opportunity. Upholding the tradition of innovation at Stanford University, he imitated the entrepreneurial spirit of Bill Gates and Steve Jobs. After graduating from medical school, he established a biotechnology company called Ambrosia, specializing in providing wealthy people with young blood transfusion to help them fight against aging.

Ambrosia was established in 2016. Its main business activity is to help the wealthy seniors in Silicon Valley to allocate young college students who are willing to donate blood. They first conduct blood type matching and infectious disease screening tests on the blood of recruited college students. If they are healthy, Ambrosia will buy the blood from the college students and sell it to blood-type matched wealthy individuals at a price of US$8,000 per liter. The company will also arrange the buyers to receive the blood transfusion treatment at an affiliated clinic (Figure 55).

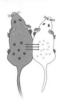

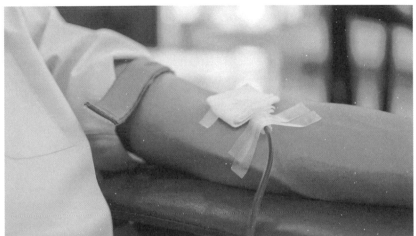

Figure 55. Customer receiving blood transfusion treatment.

Because buying blood from the Blood Donation Center to perform blood transfusion in the clinic is a legitimate medical business model in the United States, this anti-aging young plasma transfusion program does not require FDA approval.

After its establishment, all major media in the States reported Ambrosia at great length. Billionaires in the nearby Silicon Valley and around the world are all flocking. The company has developed rapidly and successfully raised the first and second round of funds, and plans to set up 20 franchised anti-aging clinics across the United States.

It is a pity that Ambrosia eventually caught the attention of FDA, who issued a warning on the company's business model on

February 19, 2019 (Figure 56). Ambrosia temporarily suspended its operations in order to avoid this public relation crisis, but after communicating with the FDA through different channels, it was back in business in 2020.

FDA STATEMENT

Statement from FDA Commissioner Scott Gottlieb, M.D., and Director of FDA's Center for Biologics Evaluation and Research Peter Marks, M.D., Ph.D., cautioning consumers against receiving young donor plasma infusions that are promoted as unproven treatment for varying conditions

For Immediate Release:
February 19, 2019
Statement From:
Commissioner of Food and Drugs - Food and Drug Administration
Scott Gottlieb M.D.

Figure 56. On February 19, 2019, the US FDA issued a warning on the business model of paid matching young blood transfusion. Source: US FDA

Ambrosia's innovative anti-aging business model has aroused considerable repercussions in the otherwise quiet anti-aging medical field. It is not the issue of rejection and infection that the FDA is criticized for, nor its treatment cost is not as unattainable as that of the stem cell industry; furthermore, it also has not caused any major medical complications to deserve the FDA warning.

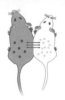

The main reason for FDA's un-proportional action is that this therapy lacks sufficient evidence on its proclaimed efficacy in aging reversal. The effect is not proven and it might lead to consumer disputes. Ambrosia had planned to raise funds to conduct clinical trials for this purpose, hoping to prove that plasma transfusion of college students is a safe and effective anti-aging treatment; unfortunately, for reasons which are not available to the public that it ended without any reasons.

If Ambrosia had gone ahead with the phase II trial, it may create a unicorn in the anti-aging industry.

Why can't the blood transfusions of college students show the definite aging reversal in organ function like Dr. Carrel's Heterochronic Parabiosis experiment?

In order to answer the question that the effect of Ambrosia treatment is not clear cut, Dr. Pan conducted an in-depth analysis of all the published papers about Heterochronic Parabiosis. He found that although Heterochronic Parabiosis experiments used an animal model of connecting one old animal to a young one. However, the age of the young mice used in each laboratory is not the same, and the results of the experiment are also slightly different.

The team of Professor Rando, which is set forth as the standard for the modern Heterochronic Parabiosis experiment, used mice that were two to three months old, but some laboratories used young mice that were four or five months old; there are no laboratory used mouse that are more than 6 months as the young mice in the old-young pair.

Dr. Pan continued his research by comparing the age of mice with the age of humans. He uses the exclusive database made available to the public by the Jackson Laboratory (which is the world's major experimental mouse supplier) and found that a two-month-old mouse is about 12 years old relative to humans, while a three-month-old mouse is 17-18 relative to humans. A mouse of 6 months in age is equivalent to a 20-year-old young human (Figure 57). In other words, the reason why Dr. Rando's Heterochronic Parabiosis conjoined animal experiment is so effective is at least partly due to the very young adolescent mice used in the old-young pair. Dr. Pan, therefore, hypothesized that: although the blood used by Ambrosia is safe and legal, it probably had exceeded the upper limit of adolescence, which resulted in ambiguous results.

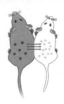

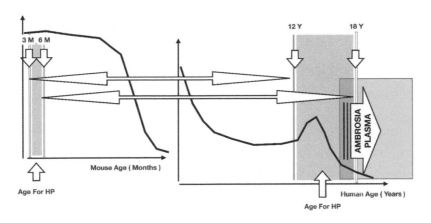

Figure 57. Comparison of the age of mice and humans. Dr. Pan research found that the young mice used in Dr. Randol's conjoined animal experiment were about 12-15 years old when converted to human age.
(Image source: https://www.jax.org/news-and-insights/jax-blog/2017/november/when-are-mice-considered-old)

21. Why Is Phnom Penh Plasma Not Feasible?

In order to solve the age-old problem of systemic aging reversal, Dr. Pan decided to search for adolescent plasma in developing countries to simulate the effect of conjoined Heterochronic Parabiosis through intermittent transfusion.

Among all the developing countries in the world, Cambodia surfaced as the optimal source of adolescent plasma. Cambodia is one of the countries with the lowest average age. Phnom Penh, Capital of Cambodia, is only three hours away by flight from most of Asia. This is very important to lower the cost of transporting refrigerated plasma internationally should the business become successful. Furthermore, Cambodian government provides a convenient visa on arrival service for visitors from all over the world to promote its tourism.

In June 2016, Dr. Pan visited Phnom Penh for the first time with the help of a friend who recently relocated to Phnom Penh. During the visit, he learned about the local regulations on the age of blood donation. After being informed that there is no strict limit, he went ahead and set up a biotechnology company called BIO-US at the landmark Hotel Cambodiana centrally located at

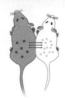

the center of the City and began to collect blood and process plasma of local teenagers.

After successfully obtaining dozens of samples, Dr. Pan was very excited and immediately contacted his anti-aging clients from all over Asia. To the surprise of Dr. Pan, however, when the client learned of the source of plasma, almost all rejected the offer due to safety concerns regarding contracting AIDS. (i.e., Acquired Immunodeficiency Syndrome).

As a result, these blood is used for research and provide the key information which led to the final solution of young plasma supply.

22. How About Artificial Plasma?

Although Heterochronic Parabiosis is the only way that has proven to quickly reverse aging in human history, however, regardless of using autologous, allogeneic or xerographic blood or plasma, there are lacking clinical trials to show its actual effects, mostly due to the shortage of adolescent plasma.

Some scientists have begun to think that although the technology of artificial blood is still immature, the use of DNA or RNA recombination to produce protein (Recombinant Protein) has become common in the field of biotechnology. If the price of protein analysis can be reduced to an extent that all the proteins in the serum of different ages could be analyzed and compared, the unique protein components in the adolescent plasma might be identified. This will allow the use of recombinant protein to manufacture them in large quantities and offered to the anti-aging clinics as a formulated drug like chemotherapy agents and total parenteral nutrition.

This approach was first taken by professor Wagers of Harvard University. Her laboratory successfully isolated a protein called GDF-11 from the blood of young mice in 2011. She also applied a recombinant form of these growth factors to conduct various experiments. Although animal experiments were mostly successful, clinical trials usually stopped after phase I trial. Its actual effects are yet to be confirmed.

Since there are nearly ten thousand kinds of proteins in human plasma, it is very difficult to identify the unique substances in young blood. Although the number of specific proteins in the young plasma might not be too many, the price of each synthetic protein is very expensive. For example, 1 mg of GDF-11 costs US$34,000. Considering supplementing three to four proteins per anti-aging treatment, the cost will quickly add up to be more than US$150,000 per injection. In addition, these proteins usually have a short half-life, so they need to be repeated in daily intervals. As a result, it costs about millions of dollars to fight aging every year!

Therefore, this kind of artificial young plasma protein formulation could not easily be accepted by the market. It will be difficult to promote. If we want to conduct a clinical trial similar to the development of a new drug to prove its anti-aging effect, a huge amount of money and decades of time will be required to obtain FDA approval. In reality, no one other than international pharmaceutical giants can afford this.

Tony Wyss-Coray from Switzerland is a professor of neurology at Stanford University School of Medicine. He was a collaborator with Drs. Rando and Conboy. Like Dr. Wagers, he wanted to find the unique protein in the young blood, so he used advanced proteomics analysis technology pioneered by Somalogic to carry out an ambitious large-scale research project.

His research team took blood from thousands of volunteers between 20 and 95 years of age, and performed quantitative analysis and statistical research on over 1000 plasma proteins, hoping to find the relationship between each protein and age.

It turns out that although there are numerous proteins in the blood and plasma, there are only four modes of association between protein and age (Figure 58).

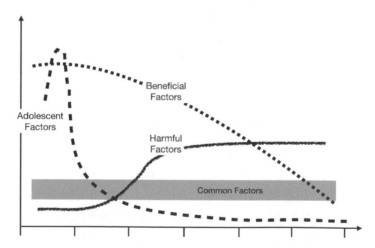

Figure 58. Patterns of protein and age association. The results of the study by Wyss-Coray at Stanford University showed that there are four modes of association between plasma proteins and age.

First of all, the concentration of most of the proteins in the blood (general proteins) are the same regardless of age. Simply put, this type of protein is responsible for daily work and has no direct relationship with the aging processes.

Secondly, there are proteins (toxin proteins) that can inhibit cellular functions. The concentration of these proteins in the blood begins to increase from approximately 20 years old, so it seems to be related to lifestyle habits; after the age of 50, the detoxification effect of human body decreases due to aging, and this inhibitory protein also increases at a faster rate, but eventually reached a plateau.

The third type of protein (good protein) decreases with age from the young age in a linear fashion, which represents the protein needed to maintain the vitality of cells.

The fourth type of protein is the adolescent protein (puberty protein). This is a small group of proteins which are responsible for the needs of the body for growth and sexual development. The concentration of these proteins are very high during puberty, but drops rapidly after the age of 17, and is not easy to detect after the age of 20.

Because it is not easy to obtain blood samples from adolescents, Professor Wyss-Coray excluded blood samples between 15 and 20 years old during his research. Since Dr. Pan had collected samples of adolescent blood in Phnom Penh, which allows him to perform analysis of adolescent plasma.

As a result, in order to simulate the changes that occur in the serum during Heterochronic Parabiosis experiment, we don't need to be concerned about the concentration of most proteins (Type one). What we need to do is to reduce the accumulation of inhibitory proteins (Type Two), while supplementing the activated proteins that are inversely proportional to age (Type Three) and unique to the puberty plasma (Type Four).

Taking the plasma of a 70-year-old person as an example, if we want to reconcile his plasma to the age of 20 years old, then we will need to do the following things (Figure 59): First, we must reduce the inhibitory protein from the plasma, next, we must increase the youthful protein, and adding small amount of puberty protein respectively.

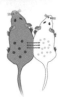

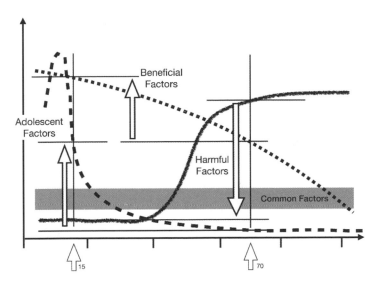

Figure 59. Comparison of serum protein between 70 and 20 years old. To reverse the age of the serum of a 70-year-old person to the age of 20 years old, the inhibitory protein in the blood must be reduced, young protein be increased, and puberty protein be increased.

In the same way, if we want to adjust the age of the serum of this patient from 70 to 15 years old, the inhibitory protein that needs to be excluded is not much different from the blood that needs to be adjusted to 20 years old. The amount of youthful protein required is also similar. However, due to the rapid decline of adolescent protein after the age of 18, a much larger amount of adolescent protein is required to adjust the client's serum age to 15-year-old (Figure 60).

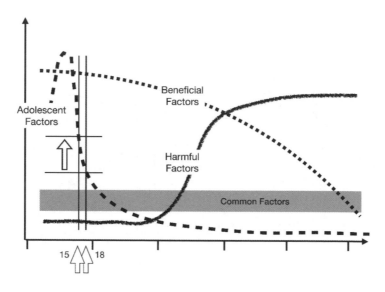

Figure 60. Comparison of serum protein between 70 and 15 years old. If the serum of a 70-year-old person is adjusted to about 15 years old, a large amount of puberty protein needs to be supplemented than adjusted it to 20 years old.

Because the adolescent protein synthesized by recombinant technology is very expensive, Dr. Pan used proteomics technology to analyze the protein components in various existing protein drugs that were currently available on the market (e.g., serum albumin, immunoglobulin, etc.) to developed formulation that can simulate the key components of natural adolescent plasma. Furthermore, he compares their activity using various stem cells with natural puberty serum and stem cell culture medium commonly used in the laboratory. It

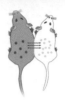

was found that artificial plasma created by blending various protein drugs can reach 85% of the activity of pure natural puberty serum and 80% of the activity of stem cell culture media (Figure 61). This resolved the biggest obstacle that prevented the translation of Heterochronic Parabiosis, and opened up the new chapter for the treatment of all-in-one intravenous Heterochronic Parabiosis. (Figure 62)

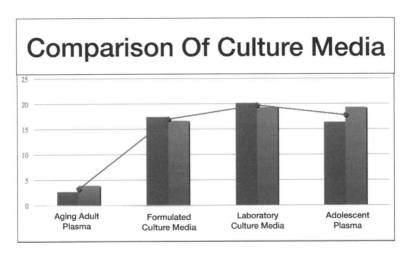

Figure 61. Comparison of the activity of the formulate serum and the adolescent serum. The activity of the formulated adolescent plasma is more than 85% of that of the natural adolescent plasma and is equivalent to 80% the activity of stem cell culture media commonly used in the laboratory.

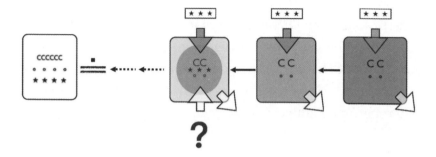

Figure 62. The innovation of producing adolescent plasma using existing protein drugs eliminates the need for actual adolescent blood which opens the gateway for performing intermittent Heterochronic Parabiosis treatment by intravenous route.

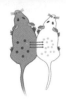

23. Why Is Stem Cells Ineffective For Anti-Aging?

After resolved the problem of the first two steps of clinical Heterochronic Parabiosis, i.e., eliminate harmful proteins that inhibit the function of stem cells, and synthesize and supplement the beneficial proteins that activate stem cells; the only problem left to be answered is the number of stem cell needed to be transplanted.

Bone marrow stem cells were discovered in the 1960s, and are commonly applied in the treatment of hematological cancer patients. Because there are cancer cells in the bone marrow, after chemotherapy eliminates the cancer cells in the patient's blood, radiation is required to remove the remaining cancer cells in the bone marrow. The stem cell transplant is required to rebuild a patient's hematopoietic system.

Although bone marrow stem cell transplantation must undergo precise matching and the process is uncomfortable, because it is not an optional treatment and there are no alternatives, the acceptance is high.

On the contrary, in the case of less severe diseases, most patients will choose a comfortable and less expensive method as compared to the bone marrow transplant, therefore applications of bone marrow stem cells in other fields is rather limited. Regenerative medicine also progressed very slowly. In fact, there were no other applications until early 1990s, when Dr. David Horowitz of the University of Pennsylvania and the Children's Hospital of Philadelphia applied bone marrow stem cells in the treatment of congenital skeletal hypoplasia (Osteo Imperfecta) and for the regeneration of skull in pediatric cranio-facial surgery.

In the millennium, the baby boomers began to enter the age of 60 and resulted in rapid changes in the population structure. The number of degenerative diseases also skyrocketed. Due to the lack of effective treatment for these diseases, stem cell biology and medicine have since gained much attention by scientists and physicians alike.

The earliest stem cell business model was cord blood banking. Its appeal is: if a baby is born with a rare disease or blood cancer, then he or she can use his or her own stem cells isolated from the umbilical cord blood or the cord itself for the treatment; to avoid the risk of rejection when using allogeneic stem cells. However, the volume of umbilical cord blood is only a dozen milliliters, and the number of stem cells in it is also limited. Therefore, in the actual clinical practice, except for two to three-

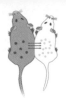

month-old babies, children who need stem cell therapy still require allogeneic (other people's) Stem cells. This abolished the advantages of autologous stem cell transplantation, the clinical application of cord blood stem cells is still very limited.

In 2002, Dr. Marc Hedrick of the University of California, Los Angeles successfully isolated mesenchymal stem cells from the adipose tissue (i.e., fat). Because a lot of people in developed countries are over-nourished, overweight, and accumulate excess subcutaneous fat in different parts of the body.

Liposuction, which is a simple and safe procedure, became very popular in the United States. Extracting mesenchymal stem cells from fat to treat local areas is like killing two birds with one stone, and quickly received public acceptance. In addition, adipose-derived mesenchymal stem cell transplantation is an autologous transplant procedure, and enjoys relaxed government regulations, and can be quickly promoted in clinical practice. It is widely used in repairing torn joint cartilage, skin rejuvenation, and hair follicle regeneration.

After the adipose-derived stem cells are successfully isolated, physicians in other fields have also found corresponding mesenchymal stem cells from the tissues in their field. For example, obstetricians and gynecologists can isolate amniotic fluid stem cells from amniotic fluid, and dentists isolate dental stem cells from the extracted tooth, etc., too numerous to mention. However, for patients who suffer from local degenerative diseases or elites who want to achieve systemic anti-aging, adipose stem cells are still the best choice due to the abundant source of fatty tissues and the ease of obtaining them.

The applications of using adipose-derived mesenchymal stem cells in the treatment of local degenerative diseases have developed more rapidly as compared to other types of stem cells. Clinicians and practitioners engaged in adipose-derived stem cell transplantation also began to expand the indication from localized conditions into systemic anti-aging.

Unfortunately, the effect of adipose stem cells on systemic anti-aging is not as clear as on local treatment. The main reason is that customers who want systemic anti-aging are generally not severely ill. Therefore, they can usually only accept stem cell transplantation using intravenous infusion, and refuse to accept the more invasive yet more effective injection of stem cells into vital organs directly.

Based on the cardiovascular anatomy, stem cells that enter the human body via intravenous injection will return to the right atrium and right ventricle, and then be sent out by the right ventricle to the lungs. Since the diameter of stem cells is three to five times larger than that of ordinary white blood cells (Figure 63), most of the mesenchymal stem cells are stuck in the

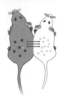

capillaries of the lungs and could not return to the left heart to be spread to other organs in the body.

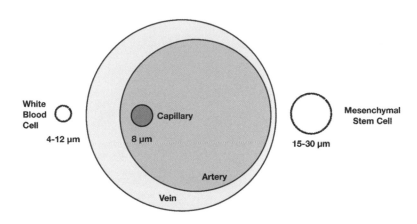

Figure 63. The diameter of stem cells is larger than the diameter of the capillaries. The diameter of mesenchymal stem cells is about 3 to 5 times larger than that of ordinary blood cells, and is larger than the diameter of the blood vessel in the lung. Therefore, most of the infused mesenchymal stem cells are stuck in the capillaries of the lung.

Another reason for the poor result of stem cell infusion in systemic aging is the high concentration of substances that are harmful to the stem cells in the aging blood. The stem cells in the laboratory are cultured in a dust-free, sterile and non-toxic environment. After being infused into the bloodstream of the patients, the stem cells cultured are soaked in toxic aging blood, and the survival rate is very low. Accordingly, autologous stem cell intravenous transfusion in clinical practice, except in a small number of pulmonary fibrosis patients, mostly failed to exert significant improvements in the function of aging organs.

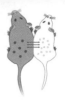

24.Since Stem Cell Transplantation Is Ineffective Systemically, Why Do We Still Do It?

Stem cells are cells that are responsible for the repair of tissues in thw human body. When there are cells in the human body that are damaged and vacancy is created, the stem cells will initiate the process of division to produce a precursor cell, and then differentiate into cells that are missing in the tissue. Therefore, early stem cell therapy is generally based on the concept of filling what is lacking, so everyone has the illusion that the more stem cells transplanted, the better the result would be.

After more than half a century of hard work by stem cell researchers, considerable progress had been made in the understanding of stem cells. Specific stem cells (such as cardiac stem cells, lung stem cells, kidney stem cells, blood cell stem cells in bone marrow, etc.) residing in various organs of the human body have been discovered and successfully cultured in the laboratory.

The most commonly found stem cell is the mesenchymal stem cells. Interestingly, it was recently found that these cells are actually not stem cells. The father of mesenchymal stem cells,

Dr. Arnold Caplan , said: When mesenchymal stem cells are in the human body, they are just a type of pericyte which adheres to the outside walls of blood vessels. Such cells are responsible for the secretion of various cytokines to regulate immune function and coordinate work among different cells in vivo.

Although scientists in the laboratory may utilize different cytokines and scaffolds to induce mesenchymal stem cells to differentiate into different types of adult cells; however, these mesenchymal stem cells will not do so after being injected into the body. Instead, it will make use of a cell migration pattern to creep out of the blood vessel to reside on the outer wall of blood vessels, i.e., pericytes (Figure 64). It will then secret all sorts of cytokines and other signaling molecules locally to influence adjacent cells or secret into the bloodstream to circulate all over the body and influence cells in the distance. (Figure 65)

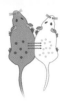

MESENCHYMAL STEM CELL WITHIN THE BLOOD

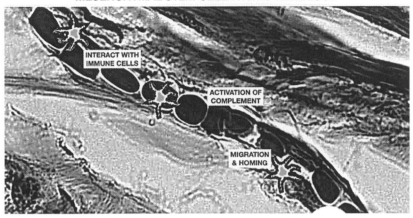

Figure 64. Mesenchymal stem cells become pericyte in the body. After the mesenchymal stem cells cultured in vitro are injected into the vein, they will slowly crawl to the outer wall of the blood vessel in a mode called cell crawling. Image source: https://doi.org/10.1186/s13287-015-0271-2

163

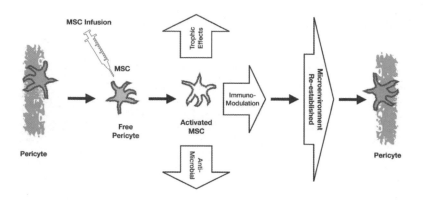

Figure 65. Function of pericytes. After the mesenchymal stem cell migration to the outer wall of the blood vessel, it will secret a variety of cytokines to affect the function of adjacent cells and other organs at the distant. Image source: https://doi.org/10.1038/emm.2013.94

In other words, after cultured mesenchymal stem cells were implanted into the body, it cannot differentiate directly into the damaged cell type to fill its vacancy. Instead, it will secret various cytokines to fine-tune the body's functions (Figure 66). Traditional concepts of mesenchymal stem cells repair damaged tissue by differentiation is not correct and should be modified. Transplanted mesenchymal stem cells exert their repair function by secreting various cytokines to activate adjacent stem cells which reside in the damaged tissue or organ.

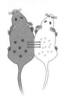

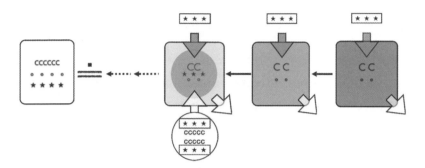

Figure 66. Repair function of mesenchymal stem cells. After cultured human mesenchymal stem cells are infused, they will not directly differentiate into damaged tissues or organs to replace the vacancy created by the injured cells. Instead, it will begin to secret various cytokines to activate adjacent and distant cells to repair the injuries.

25. How Many Stem Cells Should Be Implanted For The Best Result?

After being injected into the human body, mesenchymal stem cells become the commander of to regulate and coordinate the functions of stem cells residing in the tissue and organ. Just like you don't need too many commanders on the battlefield; the greater the number of stem cells implanted, it will cause confusion in the commanding system and even diminish the function of other cells.

Clinically, only a relatively small amount of mesenchymal stem cells is required to station in the lung (the command center), the stem cells in other organs of the body can then be directed to repair damaged tissues or to reverse the function of aging organs.

For one hundred years, after the efforts of many scientists and physicians, Dr. Carrel's conjoined Heterochronic Parabiosis was finally translated into clinical practice.

As long as the inhibitory substances in the blood are eliminated and the beneficial substances that can activate the stem cells are supplemented, the state of the serum in the human body can be adjusted into an environment suitable for the survival of stem cells. The dormant stem cells residing in various organs were then activated to repair damaged tissues and the function of the aging organ improved.

Finally, intravenous injection of trace amounts of cultured mesenchymal stem cells can be stationed in the lungs where it will secret cytokines based on the concentration of various components in the capillary. Once the interstitial environment and the immune regulatory function are optimized, the body will then gradually return to a more youthful state.

26. What Is Autophagy?

Just like there are macroeconomics and microeconomics for discussion of general and individual phenomena, physiology is a scientific discipline which studies the general phenomena of the whole body and the discipline of molecular biology and cell biology study microscopic events that happened at the cellular level.

Before James Watson and Francis Crick determined the structure of the DNA molecule in 1957, molecular biology had not yet sprouted, most of the medical research was based on physiology; after the DNA structure and related mechanisms for protein synthesis was discovered, both cell and molecular biology has flourished, allowing humans to have a deep understanding of how cells operate at the molecular level. As a result, the mainstream of medicine also became microscopic.

Dr. Carrel's research is to study the macroscopic phenomenon of aging using conjoined operations of one old and one young.

The year after Dr. Carrel passed away in 1944, there was a man named Yoshinori Ohsumi who was born in Japan, who was awarded the Nobel prize in Physiology and Medicine in 2016, 104 years after Dr. Carrel won the same award in 1912. Professor

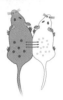

Yoshinori Ohsumi was awarded for his work of using modern molecular biology techniques to explore an extremely important microscopic mechanism called autophagy which also plays an important role in cellular aging (Figure 67).

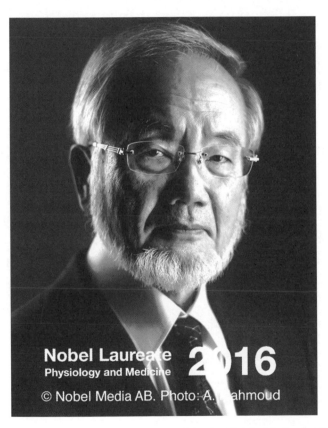

Figure 67. Dr. Osumi Yoshinori, winner of the 2016 Nobel Prize in Physiology and Medicine. Image source: nobelprize.org

Autophagy is an evolutionary conserved cellular mechanism. It is responsible to break down of mis-folded protein or malfunctioned organelle within the cells. After these substances were decomposed, the residuals of the digestion process which occurred in an organelle called lysosome, were then re-utilized for the synthesis of new proteins and organelle. Because it is a way to survive when the living subjects are lacking nutrients, it is an important life mechanism shared by most organisms (regardless of the degree of evolution).

In a nutrient-rich environment, cells will continue to absorb nutrients and expand their functions, but in a nutrient depleted environment, the cell will initiate the autophagy reaction. Cells start by separating a section of the endoplasmic reticulum, and then wrap the broken organelles and the defective products produced in the protein production process, and then combine it with enzymes to dissolve them, the substances produced are then It is used to reproduce healthy organelles and proteins (Figure 68).

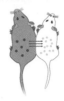

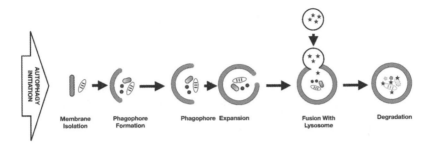

| AUTOPHAGY INITIATION | Membrane Isolation | Phagophore Formation | Phagophore Expansion | | Fusion With Lysosome | Degradation |

Figure 68. The process by which cells initiate an autophagy response. When the cell is hungry, the autophagy process will be initiated inside the cell. The cell dissolves the waste found in the cell, and the resulting material is used to reproduce new organelles and proteins. Image source: https://doi.org/10.1038/s41580-018-0033-y

Simply put, autophagy is the natural waste recycling process at the cellular level. If the autophagy reaction progresses better, there will be fewer undesirable substances remaining in the cells, and the healthier the cells will be and the healthier the cells, the healthier the organs of the human body will be. Therefore, autophagy is one of the most important molecular mechanisms for humans to fight against aging.

Since the autophagy reaction is closely related to the aging of the human body, most of the anti-aging molecular biology research is related to how to regulate the autophagy reaction. There are three regulatory mechanisms of autophagy reaction (Figure 69): First, AMPK-ULK1 (AMPK: AMP-activated protein kinase, AMP: Adenosine Monophosphate; ULK: Unc-51 Like Autophagy Activating Kinase) is a stimulating pathway for autophagy; second, mTOR (mammalian Target of Rapamycin) is a pathway for suppressing autophagy; lastly mTORC1 (mammalian Target Of Rapamycin Complex 1 or mechanistic Target Of Rapamycin Complex 1) is also a molecular pathway that inhibits autophagy.

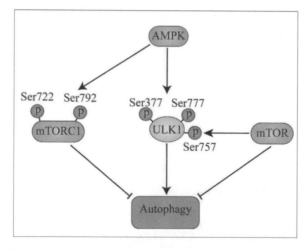

Figure 69. Three molecular regulatory pathways for autophagy. Image source: https://doi.org/10.3390/biom9100530

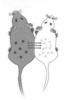

For example, because AMPK is a mechanism that stimulates the autophagy reaction, if there are drugs that can activate AMPK, it will have an anti-aging effect. On the contrary, the mTOR is a regulatory channel that inhibits the autophagy reaction, like a brake for the autophagy reaction. If the mTOR pathway is blocked, it will be like loosening the brake and the autophagy will be activated.

Both calorie restriction and Heterochronic Parabiosis initiate the autophagy reaction (Figure 70).

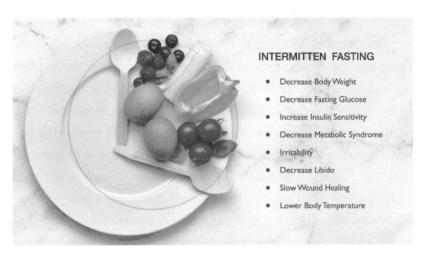

Figure 70. Fasting and Heterochronic Parabiosis both initiate the autophagy response. Image source: https://doi.org/10.1056/NEJMra1905136

In the 1930s, some scientists discovered that if laboratory animals were starved, their average lifespan would be longer and they would be less likely to get sick. Generally speaking, if the food for mice or rats in the laboratory is reduced by 30% to 60%, the maximum life span of the animal will increase by the same proportion. Interestingly, if the rats are allowed to maintain a normal food intake and then stimulate them to exercise to avoid obesity, their average life span will also be extended, but the longest life span will not increase. These results indicate that using fasting therapy is much better than relying on exercise to extend life.

Early scientists believed that the reason fasting can prolong life is that the free radicals contained in food or result from food processing will decrease with the decrease of calorie intake, so the speed of tissue damage or aging will be slower. Later, scientists noticed that the mice that were forced to reduce the calorie intake will finish their food in three to four hours, in other words, they will have a period of about 20 hours without any food to eat. Further studies revealed that their energy source will be converted from the usual glucose-based mechanism to a ketone-based metabolism. This eventually led to the discovery of intermittent fasting program that has gained popularity recently.

Scientists have further discovered that under normal feeding conditions, animals will continue to grow, and then in a fasted

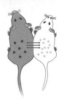

state, cells will naturally initiate autophagy to fight oxidation, improve glucose metabolism, increase stress resistance, and reduce various inflammations. reaction.

In the state of shortage of fatty acid, amino acids, glucose, and insulin, cells will inhibit growth hormone-related rapamycin target protein pathways to reduce protein synthesis and start recycling bad proteins at the same time.

In order to understand that Heterochronic Parabiosis can effectively reverse the phenomenon of aging, many scientists also use molecular biology experiments to analyze the mechanism of Heterochronic Parabiosis experiments. The results show that the autophagy reaction of cells in animal tissues and organs are activated through the molecular pathway of mTORC1 after injected with young plasma. (Figure 71)

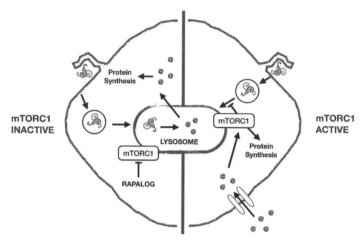

Figure 71. Heterochronic Parabiosis initiates the autophagy response. Molecular biology experiments are used to analyze the mechanism of the Heterochronic Parabiosis experiment. The results show that the tissues and organs of animals that have been injected with young plasma will initiate the autophagy reaction through the pathway of mTORC1. Image source: https://doi.org/10.1016/j.cell.2015.06.017

Through the efforts of two Nobel Laureates of Medicine and Physiology who are separated by a hundred years, mankind finally discovered a way to reverse aging that could be observed at the macro-physiological level and has a sound molecular mechanism. In addition to giving mankind a glimpse of the full picture of the aging process, this basic science also allows mankind to develop various methods to reverse aging in the future.

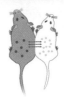

27. What Does Anti-Aging Medicine Look Like?

Looking at the phenomenon of human aging from a macroscopic perspective, it is due to the decline of the body's repair ability after the age of 50. The repair function, which is the duty of the stem cells, has become unable to keep up with the rate of destruction, resulting in tissue damage and loss of control of various regulatory functions.

From a microscopic point of view, the aging process starts through the aging of various organelles within the cell. When these organelles (such as mitochondria, endoplasmic reticulum, etc.) have problems, the waste products will begin to accumulate to make the cells bloated, they will gradually lose their regulatory functions and result in systemic imbalance, a condition called chronic inflammation. Furthermore, toxins will begin to accumulate in the blood, resulting in the decline of systemic functions (Figure 72).

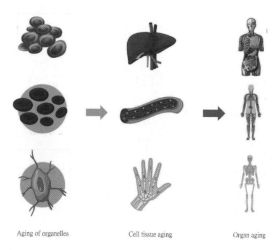

Figure 72. The propagation of aging of organelles.

If we combine the above information on macroscopic and microscopic aging, we can get a complete understanding of the aging processes and its effect on human health (Figure 73).

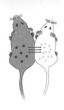

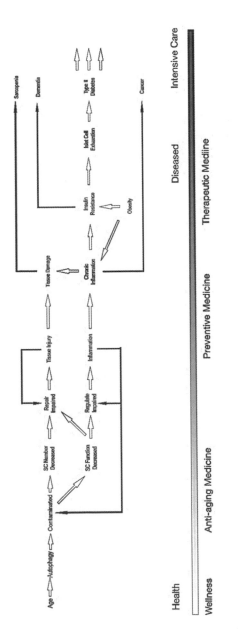

Figure 73. Road map of aging from the medical point of view.

For a relatively healthy person, who has no genetic defect, the body's destructive power and repair power are basically in a stable and balanced state before the age of 50.

Destructive power is generally related to lifestyle habits and personal psychological characteristics, while repair power is related to the number and function (biological vitality) of adult stem cells that reside in various organs. By the age of 50, the stem cells that have been resident in the organs for a long time will begin to mutate. In addition to the methylation of DNA, the organelles in the cells will also gradually become damaged.

At this time, the autophagy in the cell will be initiated to recover, dissolve, and regenerate these damaged organelles and proteins that have failed to fold properly. If there is too much waste and toxins accumulate in the cell, or if the autophagy reaction is inhibited for other reasons, the environment will be polluted and become a norm in the cell, which will certainly affect its function.

If concentration of the toxin continues to rise, it will eventually lead to stem cell damage, apoptosis, etc. resulting in a rapid decrease in the number of stem cells residing in the organs.

Under the same living habits and conditions, the repairing power of the human body is inversely proportional to the age of the human body. The repairing power of the human body is closely related to the number and function of stem cells. When the number and function of stem cells decrease, it is the beginning of aging.

When the number of stem cells decreases, the repair force will also decrease; at the same time, cytokine secretion capacity of the stem cell will also begin to improvise, and the regulatory ability of the stem cell be jeopardized.

If damaged tissues cannot be repaired in time before further damage due to reduced repair function, defects in the structure will not be healed and permanent structural defects will result.

The reduction of the regulatory function will lead to the imbalance of the immune system, resulting in the phenomenon of tissue inflammation. These phenomena are reversible at the beginning, however, if left unattended for a prolonged period of time, it will become irreversible. Long-term tissue damage will cause scarring, and long-term inflammation will result in chronic inflammation systemically.

Tissue damage can cause some structural problems, such as muscle fibrosis, degeneration of articular cartilage, etc., and finally lead to chronic diseases such as sarcopenia, joint degeneration, and fragility. Chronic inflammation in the human body can cause insulin resistance. Insulin resistance prevents the liver, muscle, and fat from responding to the insulin to absorb glucose in the blood, leading to an increase in blood sugar. At this time, the pancreatic islet cells will misunderstand that the insulin secreted by it is insufficient, they will continue to produce insulin until exceeds their load and become exhausted. The vicious circle continues until pancreatic islet cell failure and leads to type 2 diabetes.

Type 2 diabetes can be called the mother of all diseases. It can cause microvascular disease all over the body, which can lead to diseases of the cardiovascular system, chronic renal failure, and retinal degeneration. Alzheimer's disease, which is increasing rapidly with aging of the population, has also been confirmed to be related to the insulin resistance of the brain, and is sometimes considered as type 4 diabetes.

The human body is constantly being damaged by external physical forces (such as electromagnetic waves, cosmic rays, etc.) or toxic chemical substances, many mutated cells in the body are therefore being generated in a constant fashion. The body is relying on our immune system to eliminate these potentially cancerous cells. Chronic inflammation will cause the body's immune system to malfunction and allow mutant cells to escape the immune surveillance, which may eventually lead to cancer.

Conjoined Heterochronic parabiosis exerts three major functions (Figure 74): at the cellular level, it will activate autophagy to improve function of the aging stem cells; at the

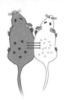

tissue level, it will re-activate the repair function and regulatory function of the stem cell; finally, at the physiological level, it can quickly rebuild and repair damaged tissues and resolves the chronic inflammation, which will reverse the function of aging organs and systems.

During the intermittent heterochronic parabiosis procedure, the first step is to exclude toxic plasma, which can immediately improve the body's macroscopic environment; Second step is the infusion of supplementary artificial adolescent plasma, just like intermittent fasting, it can activate the autophagy process to allow stem cells residing in major organs to function again. Finally, transplanted mesenchymal cells will stay in the lungs, monitor and respond to subtle changes of cytokine concentrations in the bloodstream. Altogether, the body's repair force will increase significantly. It will not only balance the destructive power immediately, but also reverse various undesirable conditions that had accumulated in the body over the time.

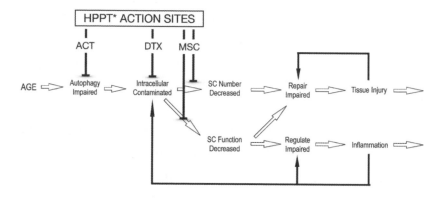

* HPPT : Heterohronicc Parabiosis Plasma Therapy

Figure 74. The function of Heterochronic Parabiosis to reverse aging. At the cellular level, it will initiate autophagy to reverse the function of aging stem cells, and then reactivate the repair and regulation functions of stem cells, so it can quickly rebuild and repair damaged tissues and reverse the chronic inflammation of the immune systems and function of organs.

From the perspective of anti-aging medicine, the three steps of the Heterochronic Parabiosis treatment address the three key causes of aging, that is, the decline of autophagy response, the accumulation of pollution inside and outside, and the insufficiency of repair and regulation functions of the stem cells. As a result, the procedure can improve from the root cause of the disease and become the fastest and most effective anti-aging program, in great contrast to most of the treatment in modern medicine which only treats the symptoms of degenerative diseases.

28. Is Heterochronic Parabiosis Scientifically Sound ?

After completing the master plan for clinical Heterochronic Parabiosis, Dr. Pan used his background as a physical chemist to analyze the chemical kinetics of the system, he calculated the clinical parameters of Heterochronic Parabiosis based on the new model he had proposed.

The total amount of bloodletting must be calculated according to the patient's Hemoglobin, Hematocrit and Reticulocyte Count; the Heterochronic Parabiosis treatment must be performed based on the volume of bloodletting and formulated replacement adolescent plasma to harmonize the osmolarity.

Using a 65 kg adult as an example, the total amount of blood in his body is about 7.5% = 5 kg, which is about 5000 milliliters. If his hematocrit is 40%, then the volume of the blood cell is 2000 milliliter, and the volume of the plasma is 3000 milliliters.

If a more precise calculation is required, the physician can use the Nadler equation to calculate the volume of plasma:

Male: blood volume = (0.3669 × height^3) + (0.03219 × weight) + 0.6041

Female: blood volume = (0.3561 × height^3) + (0.03308 × weight) + 0.1833

Or Lemmens-Bernstein-Brodsky equation to calculate:
Blood volume = 70 / √ (height and body mass index / 22)

In order to measure the effects of Heterochronic Parabiosis treatment, Dr. Pan has also established a diagnostic technique to measure the toxicity and activity of a patient's plasma with respect to the stem cells to be transplanted.

If the toxicity of the plasma in the patient's body is high, even a small amount of plasma can inhibit the growth of stem cells completely; on the contrary, if the patient's serum is not toxic, the number of stem cells will be unaffected.

At the same time, if the activity of plasma on stem cells is low, the growth rate of stem cells will also be slow; if the activity of the plasma blood were returned to the youthful state with the supplement of specific protein and hormones, the activity of plasma on stem cells will increase rapidly, and the growth rate of stem cells will also increase.

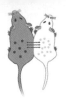

This plasma diagnostic technology allows physicians who perform Heterochronic Parabiosis therapy to control the progress of the client during the course of treatment effectively, and allow the physicians to titrate the composition in the formulation to provide best results for his client.

29. Is Heterochronic Parabiosis Being Done Clinically?

After years of planning, the intermittent heterochronic parabiosis treatment program based on Dr. Carrel's conjoined Heterochronic Parabiosis experiment was officially launched in Kuala Lumpur, Malaysia in the third quarter of 2018. Over the past three years, thousands of treatment sessions were performed on more than 1,000 patients. The results showed that the systemic effect of the Heterochronic Parabiosis treatment far exceeds the anti-aging effect of traditional stem cell transplantation.

Over the past three years, Dr. Pan's team have continuously improved the standard operating procedures, so that customer satisfaction has continuously been improved. Word of mouth began to spread and the procedure also began to attract the attention of physicians who practice anti-aging medicine in mainland China, Hong Kong, Macao, Taiwan, and Southeast Asian. In order to facilitate communication, Dr. Pan named this clinical intermittent Heterochronic Parabiosis process as MIRA (Multiple: multiple times, Intermittent: in intervals, Rejuvenation: aging reversal, Apheresis: plasma exchange) procedure to reflect on its original root and clinical essence.

Currently, the program being practiced is the 3.0 version of the MIRA procedure.

The first and most important thing is the consultation between the patient and the physician. During the consultation process, the doctor in charge should carefully record the patient's medical history and perform a thorough physical examination. The physician also needs to understand the client's expectations for the treatment. The client will then undergo a blood test and other assessment deemed necessary to assess the degree of the aging.

The part of the medical history should include the patient's chief complaint, the patient's past medical and surgical history, family history, etc., and the physical examinations should include: general condition, cardiopulmonary function, head and neck, limb examinations, etc. The blood test will usually include hemoglobin, hemolysis ratio, kidney function, metabolic function, immune function, and cancer markers, etc. Finally, the aging assessment should include the patient's muscle strength and MMSE (Mini-Mental State Examination).

The blood test report is usually available within one to two days. If the patient has no contra-indications, the treatment can be scheduled.

On the day of the first Heterochronic Parabiosis treatment, blood pressure, blood oxygen saturation, breathing rate, and body temperature will be checked in the beginning to confirm that the patient is in his or her normal condition. The nurse will implant a venous indwelling catheter and start drawing blood for serum activity and toxicity diagnostics.

The nurse will then infuse formulated plasma of choice into the vein according to the doctor's instructions with infusion pumps. During the injection, the nurse will check the patient's status every 15 minutes. After the injection is completed, the nurse will check the patient's vital signs again, and then report the value to the doctor on duty to obtain clearance of discharge from the clinic. The indwelling catheter is removed. Guests can leave the clinic after they take a brief rest in the reception area.

The nurse will call the patient to track the status and understand the reaction in the evening and the next day of the treatment. After the treatment, the staff in customer service will conduct postoperative satisfaction interviews in two weeks, and arrange post-operative consultation with the doctor.

In order to serve customers who wish to use a non-invasive method for anti-aging treatment with Heterochronic Parabiosis, the R&D team has successfully developed an oral formula that can restore plasma activity to adolescence in 2020; research has shown that this oral formula can produce a similar effect like the

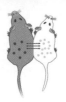

intravenous formulation. It can effectively initiate the same degree of autophagy reaction, enhance mental strength and immune function, reduce risk of infectious diseases by bacteria and viruses, and reduce the risk of cancer recurrence or metastasis.

30. Are There Any Clinical Cases In Heterochronic Parabiosis?

(1) Type 2 Diabetes

Ms. Wang from Malaysia is the earliest guest of Heterochronic Parabiosis Therapy in Kuala Lumpur. She is a very typical Southeast Asian Chinese, and speaks very mildly. Every time when she came to the presentation, she just sat quietly next to her husband. When listening to the Heterochronic Parabiosis conference for the first time, Ms. Wang quite agreed with the concept of improving diabetes by reversing the chronic inflammation caused by aging through the Heterochronic Parabiosis treatment; but there is a certain degree of suspicion. Surprisingly, Ms. Wang's husband was very supportive of her accepting this relatively novel treatment method.

Ms. Wang's husband is a senior accountant and has his own firm. The couple had been married for over 20 years. He was worried that diabetes could cause serious disease on Ms. Wang in the future. He told the consultant that his position is: as long as the treatment is harmless, has science behind the treatment, and the price is reasonable, he is willing to encourage Miss Wang to try it out.

With the encouragement of her husband, Miss Wang decided to receive treatment after two weeks of thinking. Accompanied by her husband, she had an in-depth consultation with Dr. Pan in Kuala Lumpur's office, and underwent a blood test. The results showed that her glycosylated hemoglobin (HbA1c) level was as high as 9.0, and her blood sugar before meal was as high as 250 (unit) This result surprised Ms. Wang very much and she was further determined to accept the Heterochronic Parabiosis treatment.

On the day of treatment, Ms. Wang was accompanied by her husband, arrived very early. The two were a little nervous, but also full of expectations. The course of treatment was performed by a Malaysian registered nurse arranged by a dispatching company in advance. The program was carried out according to the instruction set by Dr. Pan, and went smoothly. Miss Wang did not experience any discomfort during the procedure.

Ms. Wang said that: "I felt better immediately after receiving 150ml of serum."

She said that her husband would ask her to check her pre-meal blood sugar every morning. Originally it was around 220, and no treatment could improve it. After taking only one session of Heterochronic Parabiosis, the blood sugar dropped to about 160 before breakfast the next morning. "I was very surprised by the effect of Heterochronic Parabiosis" Wang also mentioned that the quality of sleep has become better, and some of her friends say that her face looks much younger than before and suspected that she went for plastic surgery or aesthetic medical treatment.

Since Ms. Wang's husband is an accountant, he also analyzed Ms. Wang's daily blood sugar records. He said that after the first course of treatment, blood sugar dropped rapidly for a few days, then rebounded slightly, and then began to drop again; in this way, it showed a gradual downward trend in a jagged manner. Based on the result of the first course of treatment, Ms. Wang decided to continue with the second and third courses of treatment. Her glycated hemoglobin dropped rapidly from 9.0 to 6.2, her blood sugar before meals also reduced from 220 to 120 (Figure 75). Her diabetics doctor also began to reduce the dose of her oral medication for the first over the past several years and there was no relapse.

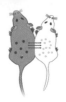

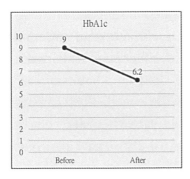
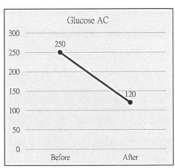

Figure 75. The blood sugar and glycated hemoglobin levels were both improved after a type 2 diabetic patient received Heterochronic Parabiosis therapy.

Although the effect of Heterochronic Parabiosis therapy for Type 2 Diabetes could be very good; Ms. Wang's case is actually quite rare. Because of the support of her husband, Ms. Wang records the blood sugar before meals and the calories intakes every day, and she takes medication on time to maintain a consistent and relatively healthy lifestyle. Therefore, the Heterochronic Parabiosis therapy can show obvious effects on her.

The case of Ms. Wang shown that, for diabetic patients in the early and middle stages, if they can improve their diet and living habits, and are willing to accept few courses of Heterochronic Parabiosis, the symptoms and signs of diabetes can be effectively controlled and improve.

Since the target of the Heterochronic Parabiosis treatment is the root cause of diabetes, which is the chronic inflammation resulting from the aging process, its effect can be maintained for at least 3 years. In other words, if the living habits of early and mid-term diabetic patients have improved, they can use this method to reverse aging to reactivate the islet cells in the pancreas, to restore the function of the islet cells to secrete insulin, gradually lower the blood sugar, and return the body to a healthy state.

(2) Presbyopia

Ms. Huang is an excellent financial officer. She once served as a spokesperson and was also responsible for the fundraising of many listed companies. Ms. Huang pays great attention to health. According to her, she strictly practices intermittent fasting and is able to maintain her body shape and weight just like when she graduated from college in the States.

Because Ms. Huang is very active in the investment community of biotechnology, she participated in a seminar about Heterochronic Parabiosis and became highly interested in this century old biotechnology. She also took the initiative to try out a treatment session.

Since Ms. Huang's experience in fundraising may need to be used to expand the business in the future, the company quickly

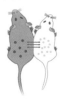

arranged a trial session of Heterochronic Parabiosis Plasma Therapy for her. Halfway through the course of treatment, Ms. Huang developed an allergic reaction on her skin. After taking an antihistamine, the allergic reaction alleviated immediately, and she was able to continue her infusion. The medical team could not help but worry that she might have some negative comments on the Heterochronic Parabiosis treatment.

Fortunately, when the customer service followed up with an interview the next morning, Ms. Huang said that she noticed something which surprised her, that is, the presbyopia that had plagued her for many years had recovered! She said that usually requires glasses to use the cell phone, however, the next morning she realized that she could read the fine prints on the cell phone without the reading glasses. When the customer service staff informed Dr. Pan about her improvement in vision, Dr. Pan originally thought it was the placebo effect and disapproved of it. However, as more and more of the clients of Heterochronic Parabiosis expressed similar reactions, the improvement in presbyopia attracted the attention of Dr. Pan, but remained puzzled.

Parabiosis is to improve the blood activity in the body by reducing toxins in the blood and increasing the beneficial substances in it. Therefore, the organs that benefit first are usually those with good circulation. Since the lens of the eye does not have any blood circulation, so that it should not have an immediate effect. After Dr. Pan discussed this phenomenon with a few ophthalmologists, and the mechanism behind this effect was revealed.

The adjustment of the focus of lens is related to aging; it is mainly derived from the muscles that adjust the focus gradually reduce the force of contraction with age; the Heterochronic Parabiosis therapy can reduce the toxins in the blood that flows through the muscles, so it could reactivate the stem cells of the muscles to repair and restore the contractility of the muscles to the youthful state, thus result in reducing the severity of presbyopia.

(3) Retinal Degeneration

In addition to being effective against aging-related presbyopia, Heterochronic Parabiosis can also be used to improve degenerative retinal diseases, i.e., macular degeneration or retinopathy by other reasons.

Mr. Li is a young man accompanied by his mother to the clinic for consultation. He was a little rebellious. His words are full of dissatisfaction with the current social phenomenon, which can be said to be a typical angry youth. During the consultation, Mrs. Li said that Mr. Li suffered from glaucoma of unknown origin, and his eyesight was impaired. She said that she didn't know the seriousness of glaucoma, so she did not take Mr. Li to see a doctor until his vision was damaged, and felt very sorry about it.

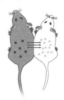

She saw an EDM on a Heterochronic Parabiosis Lecture on Facebook, and made an appointment for consultation with Dr. Pan immediately before attending the event. She wanted to know if Mr. Li's retinopathy had a chance to be improved by this treatment. Dr. Pan told her: "Heterochronic Parabiosis treatment is for the treatment of aging-related degenerative diseases. Since the vision loss caused by glaucoma can also be regarded as a degenerative disease, the condition might be indicated and there is a slight chance that it might work." Because the economic status of the family was not good, however, touched by the expectation of mother and son, the company decided to provide a session of treatment for Mr. Li at cost, to see if there was any room for improvement in his deteriorated vision.

The Li's accepted the offer. After the treatment, Mr. Li said that his visual acuity has improved and everything he saw has become much clearer. The mother also said his son was very happy with the result and willing to continue the treatment to restore his degraded vision. It is a pity that due to financial reasons; Mr. Li could not continue the treatment and was lost in contact.

Not only Lotusbio Technology Co., Ltd., but also Alkahest company in the States is interested in applying Heterochronic Parabiosis technology for the treatment of degenerative diseases of the retina. They used small molecules that could block chronokine identified in their HP platform for the treatment of aging related macular retinal degeneration of has completed clinical phase 1 and phase 2a studies. The company also said it will develop medicinal serum preparations that can control macular degeneration before 2025!

(4) Breast cancer

Cancer is one of the most feared diseases of any modern society. It has been the number one cause of death among most of the Asian countries for many years, it also has been one of the leading causes of death in Western countries where cardiovascular diseases are even more prevalent.

The incidence of most of the common cancers, e.g., lung cancer, colon cancer, breast cancer, liver cancer, increased rapidly after the age of 50. Although the cause of each cancer is different and mostly remains unclear, however, there is no doubt that occurrence of cancer is closely related to the aging process.

The primary goal of early cancer treatment is to eradicate all the tumor cells!

If the tumor has not metastasized and the patient's physical condition is in a state to undergo the anesthesia and surgery, resection is usually the first choice for cancer treatment. Surgery emphasizes the complete removal of the tumor with clear margins and lymph nodes adjacent to the tumor were also sampled. If the edge of the resection specimen or the biopsy of the lymph node during the operation contains cancer cells, the patient will then be required to receive further resection in combination with chemotherapy and or radiation therapy.

Chemotherapy relies on the rapid division and growth characteristics of cancer cells; the chemo agents are usually toxic compounds that could be absorbed by rapid dividing cells. Since chemotherapy drugs will be distributed throughout the body, during the chemotherapy, the agents will also kill a large number of healthy cells which have a relatively high division rate, at the same time, and result in various side effects.

Radiotherapy is different from chemotherapy in that it kills local tumor cells. Like surgery, the goal of radiotherapy is to completely remove tumor cells by the energy of radiation. High doses of radiation are usually required to accomplish this goal, which not only destroy normal local tissues, but might also lead to serious local and systemic side effects.

Regardless of surgery, chemotherapy or radiotherapy, the physical status of the cancer patients will be severely depleted following the therapy. Therefore,the patient's immune function, which is required to eliminate residual or circulating tumor cells to prevent local recurrence or distant metastasis, is also severed.

In recent years, many physicians have begun to wonder: if the number of residual cancer cells in the body is not very large, then it will be possible for the body to contain these residual cancer cells by its own immune function, and there will be no need to eradicate all the cancer cells. In other words, this concept of allowing residual cancer cells to coexist with the host under the supervision of the immune system, argues against the use of extreme measures to remove all the tumor cells at the expense of traumatization and reduction in immune function.

In addition to killing pathogens that might cause various infections from outside the body, the immune system also eliminates mutant cells produced in the body. Just like all major systems in the body, the aging process will also decrease the function of the immune system. The effectiveness of removing the mutant cells (cells that may turn into tumors or premalignant cells) in the body will also be reduced, and the chance of developing cancer increased.

If we can reverse aging, the immune system can be reactivated and the mutant cells would be eliminated more effectively. Therefore, the remaining cancer cells in cancer patients can also be contained, reducing the risk of local recurrence and metastasis. This is the main reason that patients who have undergone surgery and chemotherapy or radiotherapy should consider a course of heterochronic parabiosis treatment in between these aggressive treatments.

Dr. Guo is a famous ophthalmological plastic surgeon in Malaysia. Her specialty is double eyelid and eye bag surgery.

Dr. Guo loved sports since she was a child and once represented her state government for national field and track competitions. Due to the background of being an athlete, Dr. Guo has always been very conscientious about her wellness and lives a highly regulated healthy lifestyle and conducts health examinations on a regular basis.

Dr. Guo was in her forties when she noticed a lump in her breast. She immediately underwent a needle biopsy, and then underwent resection surgery to remove the malignant tumor. Because the lymph nodes near the tumor had been invaded by the cancer cells, she had to undergo chemotherapy and a series of radiotherapy afterwards. At this time, she had the opportunity to meet with Dr. Pan and become familiar with the Concept of Heterochronic Parabiotic therapy. She was in agreement with the concept of managing residual tumor cells in the body by enhancing the immune function, and became hesitant to continue with the radiotherapy after the chemo.

Since Dr. Guo is a physician, she has a complete understanding of the concept of using HP therapy to prevent and reduce the risk of local recurrence and metastasis. After some serious considerations, she decided only to continue with the hormonal therapy, which is mild and has less impact on the immune system, and postponed the more aggressive form of chemotherapy and radiotherapy as the last-line treatment in case of local recurrence or distant metastasis.

Dr. Guo met with her surgical oncologist to express her decision. Originally, her surgical oncologist did not agree and thought that doing so would jeopardize the integrity of the entire treatment. Dr. Guo was not discouraged. In addition to diligent communication, Dr. Guo also provides her surgical oncologist with relevant clinical papers for her perusal. Finally, the surgeon not only agreed with this approach, but also encouraged Dr. Guo to share this concept with other breast cancer patients with similar staging.

Different from patients with degenerative diseases, doctors must monitor the number of circulating tumor cells (CTC, which is an objective basis for the effect of Heterochronic Parabiosis treatment) of the cancer patients who are undergoing HP Therapy. The plasma formulation also requires some modification to eliminate all ingredients that might stimulate the growth of cancer cells.

The number of circulating tumor cells of Dr. Guo was 4 before Heterochronic Parabiosis treatment. After receiving three courses of Heterochronic Parabiosis, the number of circulating tumor cells dropped to 2 (Figure 76). This shows that Heterochronic Parabiosis therapy was successful in controlling remaining breast cancer cells in the body of Dr. Guo. Dr. Guo continues to receive regular check-ups and is eventually cured and freed from her breast cancer.

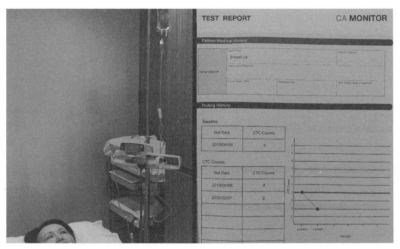

Figure 76. The number of CTCs dropped from 4 to 2 in breast cancer patients indicating the effect of HPT in containing certain cancers.

There was another episode in the process of Dr. Guo's treatment. She was undergoing hormonal therapy for breast cancer at the time of her HPT, and the body's immune function was poor. The chemo doctor warned her not to go to crowded places to avoid contracting any infection.

Due to her busy practice, Dr. Guo could only receive the Heterochronic Parabiosis therapy before the lunar year. After the serum replacement, she did not want to give up the chance to meet with her family, so she decided to take the whole family to Sabah in eastern Malaysia for the holiday. Interestingly, all the family members except Dr. Guo had a bad cold during the trip. Dr. Guo concluded by saying: "The Heterochronic Parabiosis plasma therapy must have a strong effect on promoting the immune function." She also proceeded to arrange for both of her parents to receive the Heterochronic Parabiosis treatment for the purpose of Anti-aging.

(5) Pancreatic Cancer

Pancreatic cancer is also known as the king of cancer. It is usually diagnosed at a late stage, locally advanced, and cannot be removed. At the same time, the tumor does not respond to the chemotherapy or radiation well, resulting in high mortality.

If the tumor has not expanded locally, an operation called Whipper Procedure could be performed. The operation is a major surgery. The surgeon will remove the head of the pancreas, the duodenum, part of the stomach, and the gallbladder; this generates a great burden on the patient's physical condition. However, even if the Whipple operation is performed successfully, the five-year survival rate of the patient remains approximately the same. In fact, most patients can only survive for another 6 months after their initial diagnosis of the cancer.

Mr. Zhang is the owner of a family-owned Chinese seafood restaurant in Kuala Lumpur, Malaysia. He is about 180 cm and 100 kg, works day and night, never took much care of his health and has not received a health examination for many years until his family noticed his jaundice. After which, they forced him to go to a nearby hospital for a thorough examination. During which, abdominal ultrasound revealed a tumor in the head of pancreas, and the biopsy result was pancreatic cancer.

Since Mr. Zhang is still young and the tumor did not seem to spread, the family immediately arranges for him to undergo Whipple procedure by the most famous hepatobiliary surgeon in Kuala Lumpur. The surgery went smoothly and he was discharged within a week after the operation. However, his physical condition was significantly weakened and became short of breath after a few steps, and required support to climb even a couple steps of stairs. At this time, the surgeon arranged for him to receive a full course of chemotherapy, which made the whole family very worried. In particular, Mr. Zhang's uncle feels instinctively wrong when he learns of the upcoming chemotherapy and openly objects to it.

At that time, Dr. Pan was giving a speech about Heterochronic Parabiosis in Kuala Lumpur. The uncle immediately signed up for it and discussed Mr. Zhang's case with Dr. Pan after the seminar.

Since the tumor was less than 4 cm in diameter and has been resected, Dr. Pan suspected that most of the pancreatic cancer cells should have been removed. Because Whipple is a major surgical procedure, Dr. Pan believes that Mr. Zhang's immune function was in a sub-optimal state. If chemotherapy were administered, it would cause further damage to the immune function. Apart from immediate risk of infection, the remaining pancreatic cancer cells, if there were any, might recur or metastasize and lead to a devastating situation.

Dr. Pan suggested that Mr. Zhang could consider a course of Heterochronic Parabiosis as a booster to his physical and immune conditions before deciding on the follow-up treatment for his pancreatic cancer. With the assistance of his uncle, Mr. Zhang's received his first HP therapy uneventfully. After which, his physical strength improved quickly and recovered to his pre-surgery conditions within two weeks. He received two additional treatments of HPPT and rejected the chemotherapy accordingly. It has been more than two years since Mr. Zhang's operation. His weight and vitality has been restored fully and the pancreatic cancer has not recurred. Although he is still under close monitoring for possible recurrence of the cancer, Mr. Zhang said that no matter the outcome in the end, he and his family are very grateful and satisfied with the quality of life he had in the past two years.

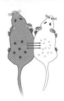

Mr. Zhang is not the only one who survived pancreatic cancer with Heterochronic Parabiosis therapy.One time, Dr. Pan went to Phnom Penh to discuss cooperation with the owner of an anti-aging clinic focused on stem cell transplant. The father of the owner was 92 years old and recently diagnosed with locally advanced pancreatic cancer. Because the father has had diabetes for many years, the rapid growth of pancreatic cancer raise the blood sugar to 600 and a conditioned called DKA (i.e., Diabetic Keto-Acidosis). DNR (i.e., Do Not Resuscitation) was signed by the family and the father was transferred to the hospice.

At this time, the owners, who were ready to give up the treatment for his father, thought of the Heterochronic Parabiosis therapy presented by Dr. Pan, decided to make a desperate move. Through personal connection, he was able to arrange for the nurse in the hospice to perform a HPPT according to the instruction of Dr. Pan. The father received infusion of Dr. Pan's plasma formulation at a rate of 50 ml per day for three consecutive days. The result seemed like a miracle. The elder man suddenly woke up and was transferred to the general ward for medical care. He was discharged two weeks later and continued to receive Dr. Pan's plasma formulation at home with the assistance of a home care nurse. The old man recovered to reach a point that he was able to stand up by himself and play mahjong with the family, similar to his condition before the current illness.

The owner expressed his gratitude to Dr. Pan's secret recipe, and he took over the distributorship of Dr. Pan's plasma in Cambodia, while using his father as examples to expand his anti-aging business in Cambodia, Lao, and southwestern Vietnam regions.

(6) Frailty and Sarcopenia

In recent years, geriatricians have paid a great attention to sarcopenia (i.e., muscle wasting in senior people). They found that the reason that elderly is prone to falls, choking, and pneumonia is closely related to this condition. Due to the reduced muscle strength, it becomes hard to maintain a good balance, so it is easy to fall; because the strength of the laryngeal muscles is reduced, there is no way to close the trachea when swallowing, so it is easy to choke. Because breathing is related to the strength of the diaphragm muscles, some of the elderlies are unable to breathe deeply due to the decreased in diaphragm muscle strength, so the lung vesicles cannot fully expand, resulting in atelectasis (i.e., alveolar collapse), which makes it easy for bacteria in the lungs to divide and grow and lead to pneumonia.

Because Heterochronic Parabiosis is effective in regeneration of muscle fibers, therefore, attracted great attention of physicians who are involved in the care of the seniors at risk of sarcopenia and sports medicine alike.

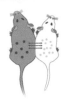

Ms. Zheng is a model and a yoga master who lives in the Bay Area. She is very sunny and pays great attention to her overall health to keep her muscle strength in optimal condition.

Once Ms. Zheng came back from the United States to visit her parents and took her personalized 3D printed face mask to the clinic of Dr. Pan for maintenance. At that time, the Heterochronic Parabiosis plasma therapy (HPPT) program was just introduced to the market by Dr. Pan. Since Ms. Zheng is a loyal customer of Dr. Pan, she decided to receive the HPPT before returning to the United States.

The next day after the HPPT, Ms. Cheng said: "my skin became very delicate and smooth, and my physical strength became very good." She was able to practice high-level yoga after walking around the streets of Taipei all day. She was fully convinced that it was due to the improvement of her muscle strength. She even said that when she went out to social with friends that night, her limited alcohol tolerance also doubled.

After returning to the United States, she continued to report the improvement through Line with Dr. Pan. She said that after the treatment, her sleep time was significantly extended, she was able to sleep from 11PM to 8AM every day soundly like a baby. At the same time, when doing yoga, the alignment of the core muscles and the time of headstand are greatly extended. According to Ms. Zheng's response, effects of HPPT could be maintained for about half a year. There are many clients who have had similar responses like Ms. Zheng.

Ms. Xu is the owner of one of the most prestigious galleries in Taipei. She is a good friend of Dr. Pan, after Brough to the attention of Dr. Pan's development, without much thinking, she paid a deposit and scheduled for the treatment. However, she forgot that the schedule of her minor gynecological surgery has been moved forward and the plasma treatment was postponed.

She was discharged from the hospital the next day after the procedure and came to Dr. Pan for incision wound care and re-schedule the HPPT. Because the injection room was free, she decided to proceed with the treatment immediately. When she got home, she started to exercise on a treadmill and ran for 10,000 steps, then continued to mop the floor without feeling tired. She said: "I was very energetic; I simply forgot about the operation which I just had." The next day, she immediately introduced several clients of hers to Dr. Pan for HPPT. All of them become long term loyal customers.

(7) Alzheimer's Disease

Alzheimer's disease has brought a tremendous impact on the social and economic status in almost every developed country. There are currently no effective treatments for this degenerative disease of the central nervous system. As more and more patients are diagnosed with the disease, the burden on the medical system also rises rapidly. The development of new drugs and new treatment for Alzheimer's disease has become the focus of major pharmaceutical companies around the world.

Alzheimer's disease is a disease strongly associated with the aging process. It is usually diagnosed after the age of 70. It is generally agreed that it might be due to the aggregation of amyloid beta proteins within and outside of the neurons in the hippocampus region of the brain, which is responsible for short term memory. If we can effectively reverse the aging process in the body, then we can delay the process that is causative to Alzheimer's disease, and there might even be the possibility of reversing this dreadful disease.

Ms. Wu is a successful business lady who owns a trading company in Taipei. She felt she had become forgetful in the past few months, went to see a neurology doctor accompanied by her longtime personal assistant. After careful examination, she was diagnosed with an early stage of Alzheimer's. Since Ms. Wu is the core of the company, her assistants went to allocate any possible treatments for her. The assistant learned about the Heterochronic Parabiosis anti-aging seminar on Facebook. Can't wait for the seminar, she contacted the clinic and scheduled a consultation for Ms. Wu.

After learning about the general concepts of Heterochronic Parabiosis Plasma Therapy (HPPT), Ms. Wu and her assistant had a brief discussion in the reception area, and decided to proceed with the treatment. After learning that the plasma used in the therapy can also be used for facial rejuvenation, Ms. Wu also bought a 3D printed face mask for her facial skin care. Because of her busy schedule, like several other female clients, she usually received the HP plasma therapy and 3D plasma facial at the same time.

After further evaluation, Dr. Pan found that Miss Wu's MMSE score was about 9 and started her treatment sessions immediately. Ms. Wu underwent 9 sessions of HPPT and simultaneous 3D facials. During this time, Miss Wu interacted with everyone in the clinic very well. The first improvement is that her original melancholic personality gradually changed and became cheerful, although her MMSE had ups and downs, it basically follows a trend of gradual improvement. As Ms. Wu's dementia gradually stabilized, Dr. Pan gradually extended her treatment interval to once every three months.

The exit examinations showed that her MMSE scores had improved to 11. According to Ms. Wu's assistant, this is much better as compared to other patients diagnosed with early stage Alzheimer's in the neurology clinic Ms. Wu went to. Most of them had gradually deteriorated with declines in MMSE scores and some even become disabled already. Miss Wu and her

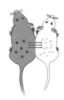

assistant are very happy that they have made the right decision to receive the HPPT.

Mr. Gu is a healthy and skinny old gentleman who has been farming in the beautiful Hualien (located in the eastern part of Taiwan) all his life. After retiring, he moved further into the countryside with his wife, while all of his children worked in Taipei. Mr. Gu's daughter once attended a seminar about Heterochronic Parabiosis in Alzheimer's Disease. It suddenly occurred to her that her mother had recently complained to her that Mr. Gu's memory is getting worse and worse, to an extent that he lost his way home twice last week, and it is getting very difficult to take care of him. The daughter encouraged the parents to travel to Taipei for a consultation with Dr. Pan.

Uncle Gu, as all the nurses in the clinic called Mr. Gu, received a blood test and a simple dementia index measurement during his initial visit. It was found that there were no problems in the blood test except mild renal insufficiency, but the MMSE dementia index was close to zero. This result surprised Mr. Gu's daughter who immediately paid out of her pocket, without consulting other siblings, to let Uncle Gu receive the first plasma treatment, hoping to slow down the deterioration rate of dementia and to reduce the pressure on her mother.

Within a month, Uncle Gu received three HP Plasma Treatments, and then took the MMSE exam for dementia again.

It turned out that there were significant improvements in his attention and calculation ability already. Most interestingly, his space orientation has returned to normal (Figure 77). His wife also stated that he stopped from getting lost in the neighborhood. At the same time, Uncle Gu's eGFR (i.e., estimated glomerular filtration rate) also increased by 15% and returned to the normal range. The family were very happy and introduced this treatment to several of their neighbors who also suffered from mild dementia or renal insufficiency. Every month, the group visited Dr. Pan clinic in Taipei for the treatment, which is a kind of domestic medical tourism.

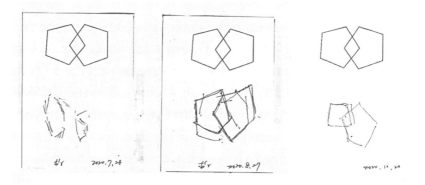

Figure 77. After an Alzheimer's patient received Heterochronic Parabiosis plasma therapy, the spatial orientation in the MMSE test improved significantly.

(8) Parkinson's Disease

Parkinson's disease, caused by abnormal secretion of dopamine in the brain, is another prevalent neurodegenerative disease. As the age of Parkinson's patients become younger in recent years, it has also received more and more attention.

Parkinson's disease is a degenerative disease of the cranial nervous system, the early symptoms are very subtle, and the general onset is around 70 years of age. Its incubation period can be as long as 10 years. The tremor of the hands and feet in the early stage is very slight and could be ignored easily. Therefore, very few patients were diagnosed at this stage. When the incubation period has passed, the patient's physical function begins to decline rapidly. Family members and patients were caught off guard and rushed to find a doctor. However, it is already past the early stage, heavy medication is required to manage the symptoms. Since drug treatment has many side effects, most patients and their family members are not compliant, and the treatment. The Results are usually not satisfactory.

Mr. Liu was an executive in a large multinational company. Soon after his retirement, he experienced intermittent tremor of hands and feet and occasional episodes of slurred speech. The family immediately took Mr. Liu to the hospital, and was quickly ruled out for stroke and brain tumor. Because Mr. Liu's symptoms usually lasted a few hours, the doctor had difficulty determining whether his problem was due to seizure or other brain problems. During further work up and repeated consultations, Mr. Liu's condition became worse.

At the recommendation of his colleagues, Mr. Liu and his family had an in-depth consultation with Dr. Pan regarding the Heterochronic Parabiosis Plasma Therapy (HPPT). The first treatment went smoothly. After returning home, he did not feel anything uncomfortable except a little groggy that night. The next morning, Mr. Liu felt that his limbs became stronger than the day before. The family also felt that Mr. Liu's mood brightened up and his articulation became less sluggish. With these positive reactions, Mr. Liu and his family decided to continue with two more sessions to complete the course. Mr. Liu told Dr. Pan that after the treatments, he could walk around the house more easily. As his speech became clearer, he also had more conversation with his family and friends. He humorously said: " I can start playing mahjong to make money to cover the expenses for the treatment ! " Although Mr. Liu's treatment was still very early, his family and friends are all excited about his improvement.

It is worth mentioning that, like many sarcopenias or frailty patients, the muscle strength of Parkinson's patients also might decline rapidly. In addition to falling and choking, which can lead to aspiration pneumonia, insufficient muscle strength can

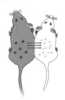

also reduce the diaphragm strength which might result in the decrease in inspiration volume and risk for bacteria or viral pneumonia.

Before the Heterochronic Parabiosis therapy, the doctor will ask them to take a measurement for FEV1 (i.e., Forced Expiratory Volume) which represents the volume of the air that the lungs can exhale in 1 second. Current data shows that if the patients combined the Heterochronic plasma therapy with breathing ball physical therapy (inspirometer) , Their FEV1 will be improved by at least 15% (Figure 78). In this way, the alveoli of the lung can be better expanded, and the oxygen exchange become more efficient; in addition to improving oxygen supply to the brain and the vital organs like the heart, the chance of pneumonia will also be reduced.

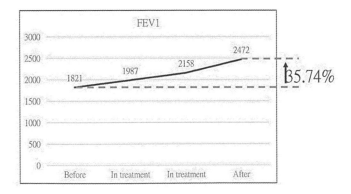

Figure 78. Patient's lung function can improve by up to 30% after receiving Heterochronic Parabiosis plasma therapy.

(9) Chronic Renal Failure

Ms. Li is an energetic elder lady in her early 80's. She was born to a family with many doctors. Her husband was a general surgeon and her daughter was an internist. She is no stranger to anti-aging treatment methods.

Her eldest daughter, Karen, was helping Dr. Pan to prepare the seminar activities of the Heterochronic Parabiosis treatment. Because Ms. Li had several chronic diseases, she encouraged her to attend the presentation. Ms. Li has always been craving for new knowledge and is willing to accept new medical ideas. After listening to Dr. Pan's presentation, she immediately forwarded her medical records to Dr. Pan for evaluation. Dr. Pan discovered that Ms. Li has a long history of Type 2 Diabetes and cardiovascular disease. She also had undergone several major operations in the past. Despite all these, her overall condition was actually quite good. In particular, her IGF-1 level was equivalent to women of 50 years old. The only thing to be concerned about is her renal function which is suboptimal. The BUN and Creatinine levels have been hovering on the verge of needing to start dialysis.

Like most people, Mrs. Li is very afraid of dialysis and pays great attention to her diet. However, her blood urea nitrogen and creatinine levels remained high. Recently, a couple of scientific publications indicated that, by simply diluting the old blood or

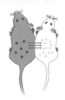

plasma, the renal function of the kidney might be improved significantly. Furthermore, since the plasma formulation already had improved the renal function of several of the patients, Dr. Pan encouraged Ms. Li to receive the HPPT.

After the explanation, Ms. Li immediately decided to proceed with the treatment. During the workup, Dr. Pan incidentally found that few of the cancer markers, AFP (Alpha Fetal Protein) and CEA (Carcinoembryonic Antigen) of Ms. Li are both elevated. Since Ms. Li just had her full health checkups, and there was no suspicion of cancer. Because chronic kidney disease may also elevate some of the cancer markers. Dr. Pan decided to go ahead with the treatment as originally planned.

After Ms. Li received three treatments of HPPT, the blood urea nitrogen and creatinine level have both significantly improved, and the renal function also increased by 30% (Figure 79). Although Ms. Li's creatinine index is still a little higher than the normal range, her blood urea nitrogen (BUN) index has returned to the normal range, and the family were relieved.

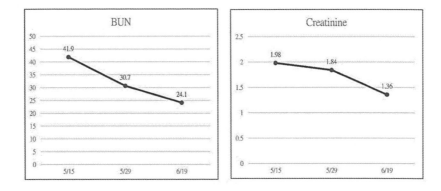

Figure 79. Renal function of chronic renal failure patients have improved after receiving HP Plasma Therapy.

Mrs. Lee began to introduce many of her friends about the concept of HP and become a community spokesperson for the procedure. What makes everyone even more happy is that after the course of treatment was completed, both of her elevated cancer indexes (AFP and CEA) have also begun to decline (Figure 80).

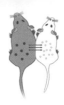

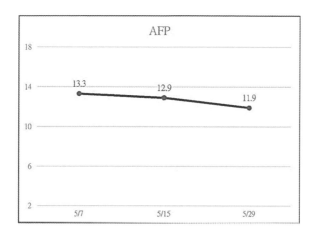

Figure 80. Cancer markers of chronic renal failure patients decreased after HP Plasma Therapy.

There was another episode in the treatment course of Ms. Li. After receiving the first two plasma therapy, she clearly felt her body vitality had increased, which made her feel excited and difficult to fall asleep. After the third treatment, Ms. Li felt a little fatigue for a few days and she was concerned. The doctor on call spoke with her over the phone and found that Mrs. Li's body temperature, blood pressure and heart rate were normal. Because the outdoor temperature was 38 degree C at that time, the doctor suspected that her fatigue was the result of a mild heat stroke from insufficient water intake. The symptoms resolved spontaneously after Ms. Li drank more water. No further treatment is needed.

Many people wonder what should be done after HPPT. Dr. Pan always said that what needs to be done is to maintain the same living habits, which means that we should not change the daily routine, nor should we change our medications. Only this could allow us to observe the effect of the HPPT objectively.

(10) Sexual function

Based on the clinical experience of Dr. Pan, who has performed thousands of cases of Heterochronic Parabiosis Plasma Therapy (HPPT), there are fundamental differences between male and female anti-aging patients. Male patients are less sensitive and have more specific needs for anti-aging, that is, the improvement of sexual function. Many male elites are very proud and confident about their achievement, but feel helpless when they experience a decline in their sexual performance.

Dr. Pan said that for these businesspeople who are very successful in their careers, they work and live a very high-pressure life. They often need to socialize heavily and it is very difficult for them to maintain a healthy lifestyle. In fact, a significant portion of them have hidden microvascular diseases, which is responsible for the decline of their sexual function and performance. Although there are oral sexual function drugs such as Viagra and Cialis on the market, because of their pride, the need for drugs to conduct their sexual performance is detrimental and unacceptable. Many of the male anti-aging

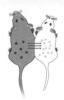

patients who come to Dr. Pan are actually seeking improvement in their sexual performance.

Interestingly, although these male patients have high expectations for the improvement of sexual function from the anti-aging program, few people openly expressed this demand to the doctor during the initial consultation. Even after the completion of the program, these patients also would not discuss the issues when they come back to the clinic for exit interviews. Instead, they often discussed frequency of their morning erections, length of sexual intercourse, and physical strength inadvertently during their conversations with the male counselors.

The same problem also occurs regarding the hair. The elites generally do not want to use oral Finasteride to maintain their hair volume. They think that if they need to rely on drugs to maintain thick hair, they will lose their pride. Of course, they also worried about the negative impact of Finasteride on their sexual function.

This shows that men's big ego centric and women's instinct to express and communicate are very different in essence.

Mr. Yang is the sole owner of an engineering company. The business is busy and very profitable. Whenever he comes to the clinic for treatment, he always works on the computer while getting the plasma infusion. As prescribed by Dr. Pan, Mr. Yang has undergone three HPPT sessions. When he came back for an interview with Dr. Pan, he only smiled and said that he felt that his physical strength seemed to have improved. But when he was leaving the clinic, he opened the chatterbox with the clinic manager, and shared various changes he has felt after receiving the therapy. He told the manager that his hair was originally sparse, but after receiving the treatment, he actually started to grow hair, and the bottom of these newly grown hairs are black in color. In addition, he also said that every time he played golf, the distance of his tee-off had increased by about 20 meters, which impressed his golfer friends.

Mr. Yang will usually end the conversation with a description about his intimate time with his girlfriend which is significant for extension in time and increase in strength and intensity. Everyone is very happy for him. Mr. Yang is an early-stage diabetes, with the help of nutritionist and plasma treatment, his glycated hemoglobin has dropped to normal range. Dr. Pan believes that if he can continue to maintain a healthy diet and go to play golf regularly, then he only needs to come back to the clinic for routine booster plasma sessions annually.

(11) Menopause

In contrast to men's attention to sexual function, women are more concerned about issues related to menopause.

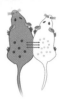

Ms. Wang is a full-time mother with two twin boys. She said that taking care of the twin is more challenging as compared with her previous jobs in financial services. She often feels exhausted. Since Ms. Wang was in her 40s when she gave birth to the twins. She had entered menopause when the twins were still in kindergarten.

Ms. Wang's financial situation is quite good. In order to have the physical strength to take care of the boys, she began to undergo HP plasma therapy (HPPT). After the first treatment, Ms. Wang immediately felt some physical enhancement, at the same time, her presbyopia also improved.

For most patients, it usually takes one month to complete the first three plasma replacement sessions. Due to the busy schedule of taking care of the twin, Ms. Wang could not receive the treatment on time. It took her 5 months to complete what normally took one month. Interestingly, one month after the first course was completed, she noticed her menstruation had started again.

Ms. Wang said that she never took any supplements for her menopause. Due to the concern of other gynecological diseases, Dr. Pan demanded Ms. Wang to undergo a full examination by her gynecologist. The result was completely normal.

Miss Wang told her gynecologist about the phenomenon of menstruation after menopause, which surprised her as well. Her gynecologist said that if there are more cases, maybe women in the early menopause can become pregnant with the help of HP plasma therapy, which will indeed be a breakthrough in medicine.

(12) Skin and Hair

As far as the body is concerned, men are more worried about their sexual function, while women are more worried about the menopause. In terms of appearance, men are more concerned about their hair, while women are more concerned about their facial skin.

After a few HP plasm sessions, almost all female patients told the clinic manager that their skin became smoother than before, the wrinkles were reduced, and their aging spots disappeared. Since most of the patients who came to Heterochronic Parabiosis therapy were to improve their health in the first place, they were very happy to have such "side effects". During the outpatient clinic, we often heard patients describe how their friends mistakenly thought they had undergone plastic surgery or aesthetic procedures. This indicates that, although HP plasma therapy is a treatment designed to improve the function of aging organs in the body; however, the plasma infused could also effectively rejuvenate the appearance of the clients from inside out. This can be described as the reverse transdermal Heterochronic Parabiosis process.

In recent years, hair care has gradually replaced facial care as the focus of many aesthetics clinics. This is because the rejuvenation effects of a thick and full hair and youthful hairline is not less than what could be accomplished by improvement in crow's feet and nasolabial fold.

Although the thickness and color of the hair vary significantly with pressure, external environment, and diet habits, compared to before the treatment, the hair of HP patients usually becomes darker and thicker. The diameter and density of the hair both increased under microscopic examination.

The improvement of hair resulting from HP plasma therapy has a unique characteristic. For a patient who originally had gray hair, the roots of the new grown hair after the plasma treatment will appear black. If the patient has the habit of dyeing their hair, the hair on his head will show a peculiar "black and white and black" zebra-like phenomenon. In other words, the black color at the distal end is caused by the dyeing of the hair, the white hair in the middle is hair growth after dyeing the hair but before the plasma therapy. The black hair at the bottom or proximal end are growth of young and black hair after the plasma therapy.

Heterochronic Parabiosis is a complete anti-aging program. It uses three simple steps, namely: excretion of toxic substances from the aging plasma, replenishment of factors from young plasma, and transplantation of small amounts of stem cells to rejuvenate the body. It can not only reverse the function of aging organs to restore youthful vitality, but also rejuvenate the appearance by improving the density of hair and skin.

(13) Weight loss

Ms. C is the consultant of Mira Clinic in Kuala Lumpur, Malaysia. Although still in her 20's, she has been working for a long time and has been married for several years. As a result, she appears to be quite mature compared to most women of her same age. Because Ms. C is the best consultant in the clinic, her attending physician took her to travel to Hong Kong and Taiwan as a reward for her hard work. Since her attending physician is Dr. Pan affiliation, Ms. C accompanied her to meet with Dr. Pan's clinic in Taipei for a business meeting. During casual conversation, Ms. C said that she was very satisfied with her current work and life. The only thing that bothered her was that her weight had never declined after undergoing various weight loss treatment programs. She overheard Dr. Pan mentioning HP plasma therapy could reverse aging and casually asked Dr. Pan whether HP plasma therapy could reduce her weight by increasing her baseline metabolism.

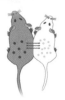

Dr. Pan thought for a while and said that: There are several types of obesity. Most are related to living habits and genetics, and the other is related to aging and decrease in metabolism. Since HP plasma therapy was originally designed for the treatment of aging-related diseases, and Ms. C is still quite young, HP plasma will not be able to improve her weight problem. Ms. C was quite disappointed after hearing Dr. Pan's opinion. At that time, the attending physician stated that in order to reward Ms. C for her outstanding performance, she decided to treat her for one session of plasma therapy. Dr. Pan could not help but agree with the request.

Ms. C returned to Kuala Lumpur with her attending physician the day after the session. Since Dr. Pan never thought that the plasma could be used to improve the weight problem of young people, and eventually forgot about it. Approximately 6 weeks later, Dr. Pan went to Kuala Lumpur to give a speech and happened to meet Ms. C again, but she was almost unrecognizable. Me. C told Dr. Pan: After her return to KL, she started the intermittent fasting diet program, which might be due to the synergistic effect of intermittent fasting and HP plasma therapy, she lost 6 kilograms of weight (from 55 Kg) in the past 6 weeks. The circumference of her waist reduced to an extent that all of her clothes must be repurchased!

Although the weight loss effect of combined HP plasma therapy and intermittent fasting was amazing, Dr. Pan still believes that

HP plasma therapy is a technique for treating aging-related diseases and can only be used to improve weight gain resulting from aging metabolism. For the young people, the best way for weight reduction is still diet and exercise. Of course, Dr. Pan is very happy with Ms. C's weight loss result.

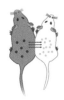

31. Are There Any Clinical Papers On Heterochronic Parabiosis?

(1) What is evidence-based medicine?

In recent years, the markets of most industries, e.g., semiconductor, internet, social media, energy, etc. are dominated by multinational companies. At the same time, the tsunami of population aging has also arrived, this provides a new frontier and opportunity for almost all small and medium enterprise companies and entrepreneurs all over the world. All sorts of companies have moved forward to establish a link with the senior related industries.

The pharmaceuticals and supplement companies are trying to develop anti-aging pills and supplements; cord blood banks and stem cell cultivation companies are trying to set up more and more storage facilities as well as translate stem cells and their derivatives into various cell therapy and regenerative biologics. Almost all major research universities have also begun to encourage university professors to take leave to translate their research into medicine by setting up biotechnology companies. The SPA and cosmetics, likewise, also begin to develop various new products using biotechnological related ingredients to take advantage of this anti-aging trend in consumer markets.

In the past few years, as social media like Facebook, IG, Twitter, Tik Tok become more and more popular, advertising marketing is no longer exclusive to large companies; companies or individual studios that have just started can carried out marketing promotion on a much smaller scale, (such as: WeChat business, internet celebrities, etc.) The propaganda methods of these self-employed or small-scale companies are very agile, and the authorities are not easy to ensure or manage the competency. As a result, social media is full of messages that are exaggerated or even dangerous. The people become tired under the bombardment of information, become unable to distinguish whether these statements are true or false, and easily be misled. It also creates loopholes in the management and control of the competent authorities in protecting the health and welfare of consumers.

These aging-related products are related to personal health and control or treatment of diseases. If these products cause physical harm or delays in treatment, it will not only decrease the effect of treatment, but may also result in irreversible consequences.

To allow consumers to quickly distinguish the reliability of the information provided by manufacturers or service providers related to the healthcare, a group of physicians began to advocate a movement called Evidence Based Medicine from year 2000, hoping to classify all clinical papers based on its credibility to give doctors a better guideline in their practice of medicine.

From low to high credibility, the basic science and clinical research or publications can be first divided into three categories: cellular experiments, animal experiments, and clinical trials (i.e., human experiments).

The simplest experiments are carried out in the laboratory using a variety of cells, and the results of these experiments are used for molecular biology or cell biology research. Although humans are composed of cells, the performance of laboratory cultured human cells and cells of the human body, is very different. If the physicians treat the human body according to the results of cellular experiments, it might expose their patients to a great risk, so the reliability of the results obtained by the cell experiment is the lowest.

Next level of experiments are the animal experiments. Traditional animal experiments usually start with the mice, followed by medium-sized animals or larger animals, and primates respectively. Due to the increase in awareness of animal protection groups, most animal experiments with the exception of mice have become harder and harder to obtain approval from the animal experiment ethics committee. As a result, most of the published animal experimental results are based on laboratory mice.

The weight of the mouse is less than 1/200 of the human body. The complexity of the mouse gene and mouse protein is also much simpler than that of the human. Therefore, except for the few evolutionary conserved mechanisms, such as autophagy, the results of the mouse experiment are far from enough to reflect what happened in the human body. Results of mouse experiment cannot replace the importance of clinical trials (i.e., human experiment).

The U.S. Food and Drug Administration once stated that 92% of the drugs that are proved to be safe and effective in animal experiments have failed to prove its results in clinical trials. This implies that more than 90% of the results of the studies in animal experiments are different from the results of clinical trials. In the worst case, the results are even opposite. If you follow the results of animal experiments and let people begin to use related drugs or receive related treatments, the risk is quite high, and the effect will definitely not be as expected. The odd of positive correlation is merely 8%.

Although many companies or manufacturers often use the results of mouse experiments to promote the effects of their products or treatments, if they want to proclaim its clinical

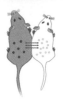

effects and FDA approval, only the results of human experiments should be used.

Generally speaking, the evidence of human experiments can be divided into five levels (Figure 81). The higher the level, the higher the credibility, and the lower the level, the lower the credibility. In recent years, due to the emphasis being placed on the importance of evidence-based medicine by the medical professionals, almost all the journal articles related to the human are required to follow the guidelines imposed by the ethics committee of the IRB, i.e., institutional review board. They will then be classified based on its credibility to various levels of evidence by the peer review committee.

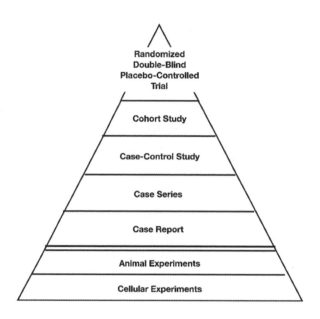

Figure 81. Human experiments can be divided into 5 levels in evidence based medicine. The higher the level, the higher the credibility; the lower the level the lesser the credibility.

The lowest level of clinical trials is called Expert Opinion (Level 5). Basically, it is the report of a single clinical case by a specialist in the relevant medical discipline. The next level of human clinical level is called the case series (Level 4), which is the result of analysis or comparison by physicians or experts in related fields on consecutive or related cases.

The following levels are: Case-Control Study (Level 3) and Cohort Study (Level 2). The former observes the difference between patients receiving treatment and those who do not receive treatment; the latter observes the effect of treatment and long-term follow-up of its results.

The highest level of clinical trials (Level 1) is the Randomized Double-Blind Placebo-Control Study. This type of clinical research is the most reliable clinical trial. The physician conducting the experiment will strictly regulate the standard of patients participating in the study, and then randomly divide them into the experimental group or control group. The experimental group receives the treatment whose effects are studied by the investigator, and the control group receives a placebo during the entire period of the experiment. No one can predict the results of the experiment during the study period unless there are major incidents, e.g., death of a subject, etc... The results of the experiment will be announced after the standard operating procedures of the entire clinical trial are completed and all the data analyzed according to the proposal. This is commonly known as blindness.

Although the evidence level of clinical trials could be clearly defined, large scale randomized double-blind placebo-control clinical trials are used as the basis for the development of most new drugs, however, not all of the medical treatment can be assessed by this highest-level standard. For example: it is very difficult for plastic surgeons to use the contra-lateral side as the control to provide evidence for the effect of the experimental side in a double-blind fashion.

Generally speaking, only cases or studies above it (Level 4 included) could be used as the clinical guideline. In other words, the minimal requirement for a study to be used as a clinical guideline is Level 4 of Evidence, which is Case Series.

In recent years, in order to promote their business, MLM companies engaged in anti-aging health supplements or skin care products have begun to arrange users to share their user experiences at their explanatory venue, hoping to increase the confidence of participants on their products. However, this kind of commercial case sharing does not belong to the scope of clinical studies, nor is it in line with the spirit of animal experiments; at best, it can only be regarded as a means of commercial marketing and has no clinical significance.

Without knowing the importance of evidence based medicine, some patients might abandon their medical treatment and opt for the MLM products. This results in loss of early treatment opportunity and leads to unfavored outcomes, many legal disputes, and waste of social resources.

We will examine scientific publications related to heterochronic parabiosis by the order of animal experiments first, followed by

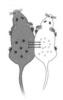

clinical trials in order of increasing level of evidence respectively.

(2) Evidences Of Heterochronic Parabiosis

31-1 Animal Experiments Related to Heterochronic Parabiosis

Since Dr. Rando restarted animal experiments on Heterochronic Parabiosis in 2005, many scientists have developed their own research protocol to mimic conjoined Heterochronic Parabiosis in order to study the effect of aging and to develop anti-aging treatments or technologies.

Although many people intuitively think, transfusion of young blood might replace the need for conjoined Heterochronic Parabiosis, research works on this approach was not published until 2014 when Tony Wyss-Coray of Stanford University published their result of intermittent Heterochronic parabiosis on the neuron of central nervous system. During his experiment, he injected the old mice with 100 microliters of young blood for 8 times within 3 weeks of time, and the observed aging reversal effect was like what was observed in conjoined Heterochronic Parabiosis.

The effect of blood sharing that occurs during the conjoined Heterochronic Parabiosis experiment is not simply the infusion of beneficial substances of the young blood into the old animal. In 2016, Dr. Irina Conboy published a paper in Nature, which explored the possibility of inhibitory effects of old blood on the function of young organs. It turns out that the inhibitory effects of the harmful substances in the old blood are far greater than the beneficial effect of beneficial substances in the young blood on the function of the old organs.

Since the blood exchanged by the young and old animals still contains a small amount of hematopoietic and mesenchymal stem cells, in a broad sense, some of these stem cells were also exchanged when performing the Heterochronic Parabiosis. Arguably, intravenous stem cell infusion might also be regarded as part of the Heterochronic Parabiosis procedure.

Just like the Heterochronic Parabiosis model established by Dr. Pan, the science of chemistry indicates that to successfully replicate the effect of Heterochronic Parabiosis and quickly reverse the aging phenomena, one must follow the three steps of removing toxic substances, adding beneficial substances, and replenishing insufficient cells in order. Therefore, whether it is simply removing harmful substances, or infusion of young blood, or intravenous infusion of stem cells, it is only a part of the Heterochronic Parabiosis process and could not reflect the whole spectrum of effects exerted by Dr. Carrel's original conjoined experiment. Likewise, any of these clinical treatments alone can only reflect a part of the full spectrum of clinical effect

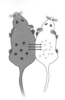

that might be produced by a combination of procedures that might simulate the conjoined Heterochronic parabiosis more accurately. This delays the time for humans to achieve the goal of reversing aging. Dr. Pan's model also laid down the theoretical foundation for clinical Heterochronic Parabiosis in the future .

31-2. Clinical studies related to Heterochronic Parabiosis

A. The addition of beneficial substances.

Just like using parabiosis (i.e., connecting two animal to live together) to study various physiological or pathological conditions might be traced as far back as Paul Bert in 1864, the transplant of tissues might be dated back even further as cited in various plastic surgery literatures.

Dr. Carrel of the University of Chicago, however, should be credited to have broken the field of parabiosis and transbiosis in his years served in the Department of Surgery at the University of Chicago between 1904 and 1906.

Carrel's work had inspired Dr. Niehans of Switzerland to develop the La Prairie therapy (i.e., the use of extracts obtained from various organs of near term fetal sheep, through intramuscular injection, to allow customers to restore youthfulness) and Japan's injection made of extracts of human placenta.

Unfortunately, both Dr. Niehans and the Japanese placenta companies (Laennec and Melsmon), due to the unknown reasons, only made very limited amount of objective evidence (e.g., medical records for finding in physical examination and/or serological test results from a third party) made available to the public. Although they both claimed to have many satisfied customers, however, both fell short to convince most of the physicians and scientists. Their works might be regarded as pioneering in the translation of findings of aging reversal observed by conjoined Heterochronic Parabiosis, but could not represent modern scientific and clinical applications of the current treatment programs based on the Principle of Heterochronic Parabiosis.

Ambrosia, is a biotechnology company established in Silicon Valley in 2014, has been frequently reported by all major media in recent years. Their business model is to create revenue by pairing Silicon Valley tycoons with college students from nearby universities, and then regularly transfuse their blood. Although the founder, Dr. Jesse Kamazin, had claimed that young blood can make people feel much younger, however, simple transfusion of ABO-paired blood from college students, seems to result in ambiguous clinical findings. The results of clinical trials conducted by Ambrosia were never published or made available to the public for examination. Ambrosia received FDA warning at the end of 2019 for the risks of rejection and infection embedded in as well as unproven results proclaimed by their program. Ambrosia quickly suspended their business. Although Ambrosia had been back in their business in 2020, however, had since been regarded as a risk taker in the lucrative anti-aging industry.

Different from Ambrosia's strategy of entering the anti-aging market aggressively, members of Prof. Rando's original Stanford team, who helped in facilitating the resurrection of Heterochronic Parabiosis in aging researchers, have taken a more conservative approach.

Professor Amy Wagers at Harvard University, and Prof. Tony Wyss-Coray at Stanford University, both began their commercialization process by analyzing the proteins in the young blood. In the hope of finding substances that are beneficial in reversing the function of aging organs. Wagers' laboratory has isolated a protein called GDF-11. After several years of animal experiments, it has finally entered phase I and II of human clinical trials recently. At present, it has entered the second phase of clinical trials for the treatment of congestive heart failure.

The practice of the Wyss-Coray laboratory is different from that of Dr. Wagers. The former's laboratory believes that the beneficial substances in the blood of young people should be a battery of proteins. They recruited 4263 volunteers between the ages of 18 to 95. The blood is analyzed for 2925 kinds of proteins, hoping to find a protein compound that can reverse aging. They also use molecular weight to categorize different batches of beneficial substances (Fractionated Plasma) and use them as novel biologicals to conduct clinical trials. Several different artificial formulations have been developed, and several phase 1 and phase 2 clinical studies are underway.

In Texas of the United States, Dr. Dian Ginzberg (Obstetrics and Gynecologist), Dr. Igor Cherches, and Dr. Eddie Patton (both Neurologist) had established a functional medicine clinic called Ginstitute to provide young plasma treatments. They used fresh frozen plasma donated by young people in the blood bank as a source of beneficial substances, and received IRB approval to perform clinical trials on Parkinson's disease and multiple sclerosis, among others. This allows patients of the above-mentioned diseases to receive young plasma exchange under the umbrella of IRB permission.

B. The removal of hazardous substances.

Although the importance of removing toxins in the blood for reversing aging was not confirmed 2016 by Dr. Conboy , however, the treatment of removing toxins from the body has been practiced in clinical medicine for many years. From the early folk therapy such as cupping and bloodletting in traditional Chinese medicine to the more recent colorectal hydrotherapy, enzyme-based colon cleansing supplement, and the use of

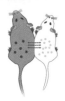

intravenous EDTA. Finally, plasma exchange, which is commonly used to treat some of the viral infection diseases of the nervous system, also started to be used as a dazzling method for eliminating toxins in plasma as an off-label application in anti-aging medical practices.

Although chelation therapy is a well-established method of detoxification, like La Prairie therapy and Placenta Injections, there are very limited publications available until very recently. In Taiwan, Yang Ming University, in collaboration with physicians from the Veteran Administration Hospital and Kaohsiung Ruan General Hospitals, published a paper on the combined use of antioxidant supplement and EDTA chelation therapy in the treatment of cardiovascular disease of patients with excessive lead or cadmium in their bodies. It was found that the heavy metals in the patient's body decreased significantly after receiving the treatment for three months, while the number of precursor cells of the cardiovascular endothelial cells and the flow rate as well as degree of expansion of the cardiovascular system would also increase significantly. These results indirectly confirmed that chelation therapy is effective in treating cardiovascular diseases of patients contaminated with certain heavy metals.

C. Combined procedure that simulates The Entire Heterochronic parabiosis.

Just like transfusion of young blood, removing the toxins in the plasma itself can not reflect the full picture of conjoined Heterochronic Parabiosis. Therefore, Dr. Pan suggested that clinical Heterochronic Parabiosis programs should include detoxification, supplementation of beneficial substances, and transfusion of insufficient stem cells. Except for younger patients (for Heterochronic Parabiosis therapy) or in better condition than people of the same age, the number of stem cells in their body has not begun to decrease, transplantation of stem cells is not justified and can be omitted. In other words, Heterochronic Parabiosis treatment can be divided into two types, one is a three-stage Heterochronic Parabiosis treatment that is suitable for older ages or patients in poor physical or medical conditions; the other is a two-stage procedure for patients who are younger in ages or in better conditions.

To the best of our knowledge, the concept of two-stage clinical Heterochronic Parabiosis was proposed by Dr. Dobri Kiprov in 2013. Dr. Kiprov received funding from the National Institute of Health to conduct postdoctoral research in clinical immunology and immunopathology at Massachusetts General Hospital of Harvard University, and became the first specialist in Plasmapheresis (i.e., washing blood) in the United States. He published a theoretical paper in the Journal of Clinical Apheresis called "Intermittent heterochronic plasma exchange as a modality for delaying cellular senescence—A hypothesis". Because of the aging population, there are more and more degenerative diseases, which has also caused a huge economic burden in every developed country. However, there is a lack of methods to treat these degenerative diseases. Since conjoined Parabiosis cannot be performed in the real world; therefore, he hypothesized that the FDA-approved plasma exchange treatment might replace the need of conjoin surgical procedure in clinical settings of Heterochronic Parabiosis.

Dr. Dobri also stated in the American Society for Apheresis's keynote speech in Denver that the use of plasma exchange to eliminate harmful substances and then supplement beneficial substances may delay aging or even reverse aging. Dr. Dobri also proposed that there are two options to supplement the beneficial substances in the plasma, i.e., fresh frozen plasma from the blood bank or serum albumin and immunoglobulin products from pharmaceutical companies. Although Dr. Dobri's hypothesis has not been translated until 2020, his thoughts have provoked a lot of inspiration for the growing number of anti-aging physicians worldwide.

It was unclear whether it was the influence of Dr. Kiprov. Grifols, one of the world's largest serum pharmaceutical companies, became interested in the use of serum albumin and immunoglobulin to treat aging-related degenerative diseases around 2010. After decades of hard work, they have conducted Phase I safety studies and Phase II clinical studies for patients with Alzheimer's disease in Europe and the United States.

According to Grifols, there is a general consensus regarding the main cause of Alzheimer's disease is insulin resistance caused by chronic inflammation and the precipitation of called Aβ1-42 and Tau proteins in the hippocampus of the patients, which causes structural damage and short-term memory loss.

Scientists at Grifols Company believe that if healthy serum albumin and immunoglobulin are injected into the blood, on the one hand, immunoglobulin can control the inflammation of the blood and reduce protein precipitation. On the other hand, serum albumin can absorb disease-causing harmful proteins to adhere to its clean surface (similar to the effect of sponge) and then be excreted from the body through plasma exchange procedures. In this way, the precipitation of abnormal proteins in the brain can be reduced and thus decrease the rate of deterioration of Alzheimer's patients. (Figure 82)

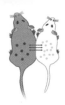

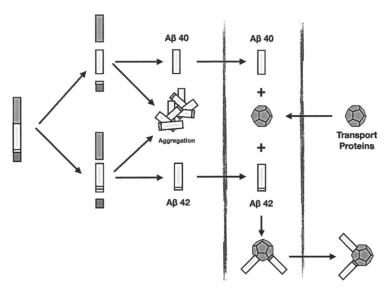

Aβ 40	Aβ 40
Aggregation	Transport Proteins
Aβ 42	Aβ 42

Figure 82. Infusion of healthy serum albumin and immunoglobulin can control the blood's inflammatory response, allowing disease-causing harmful proteins to adhere to a clean surface; they could be excreted from the body through plasma exchange, thereby delaying the progression of Alzheimer's disease. (Image source: https://doi.org/10.1016/j.trci.2019.01.001)

Grifols spent multi-million dollars to conduct multi-center clinical trials in Europe and the United States. A total of 22 medical centers in the United States and 19 medical centers in Spain participated. In their clinical trials, they examined nearly 500 patients with mild or moderate Alzheimer's disease who undergo plasma exchange on a regular basis to eliminate toxic substances in the blood and receive supplemental serum albumin and immunoglobulin.

They divided all clinical trial patients into four groups, namely 5% and 20% serum albumin ± immunoglobulin. All of the treatment courses are 14 months. For the first six weeks, each patient will receive plasma exchange once a week, and the remaining 12 months will receive plasma exchange once a month.

The results of clinical trials of Grifols Company show that if MMSE is used to track the deterioration of Alzheimer's disease, and regular plasma exchange and serum albumin and immunoglobulin injections are given; a reduction of 71% of the rate of deterioration of Alzheimer's disease patients can be achieved. (Figure 83) This is great news for tens of millions of Alzheimer's patients worldwide. Unfortunately, plasma exchange requires expensive equipment, and the cost of immunoglobulin is very expensive; at present; No company is willing to invest and conduct the last phase of the clinical trial.

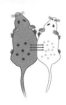

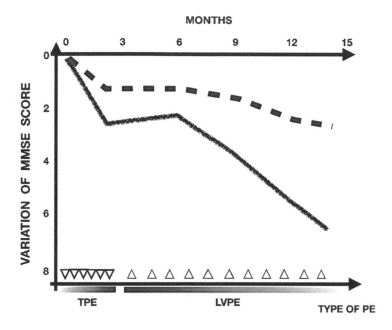

Figure 83. The results of clinical trials show that regular plasma exchanges with HSA and IVIG supplements can delay the deterioration of Alzheimer's disease patients by 71%.
(Image source:
https://www.prnewswire.com/news-releases/grifols-demonstrates-a-significant-reduction-61-in-the-progression-of-moderate-alzheimers-disease-using-its-ambar-treatment -protocol-300738956.html)

32. What Is The Impact of AMBAR Trial?

Due to the success of the AMBAR clinical trial, laboratories across the United States began to bring their Heterochronic Parabiosis related experimental results to clinical trials.

Similar to Alkahest, Professor Katcher of the University of Alabama and Professor Horvath at the University of California, Los Angeles collaborated to use Fractionated Plasma to reverse the function of aging organs. Different from other companies, because Professor Horvath has the experimental technology to directly measure the degree of cell aging by using methylated DNA,their experiments clearly indicated that the age of cells in the aging tissues can indeed be reversed after plasma treatment.

Professor Conboy, who proved that old blood is inhibitory to the organ functions, also continued to advance towards clinical trials. Unlike other laboratories, she believes that the role of blood toxins plays in the aging process far surpasses the positive effects of beneficial substances. Based on which, she is more inclined to develop technologies that can discharge toxic substances in the blood more effectively. She collaborated with Dr. Kiprov, who proposed a two-stage Heterochronic Parabiosis, and found that after the toxins in the aging blood are eliminated from the body, if simply replaced the volume loss with low

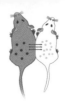

concentration serum albumin of 5% to maintain the osmotic pressure, it can achieve the same or even better reversal of the aging organs in all three germ layers of animal tissues. She also named this plasma dilution procedure as "Neutral Blood Exchange" (i.e., NBE) based on the chemistry of what happened in the process.

Since plasma exchange is a technology already approved by the FDA, they immediately took advantage of the shortcut and proceeded to Phase I and II clinical trials after the surprising result of the dilution therapy with albumin after plasma exchange in 2020.

33. Is Transplantation Of Stem Cells Necessary To Simulate Effects Of Heterochronic Parabiosis in Clinical Setting?

Because the old blood is toxic, if one infuses autologous or allogeneic mesenchymal stem cells cultured in vitro into the body through an intravenous route it will result in a very low survival rate. Only a small part of the cells will be trapped in the capillary of the patient's lungs and become pericytes of the blood vessel. From where, if adapted to the toxic plasma environment, they will exert system effect by secreting various cytokines based on the type and concentrations of various chemicals detected in the plasma.

Because the survival rate of stem cell transplantation is very poor, those who want to verify the systemic anti-aging effect of stem cell transplantation intuitively jump to the conclusion that the larger the number of implanted cells the better the effect. This misconception drives the cost of stem cell transfusion higher and higher, and resulted in many consumer disputes.

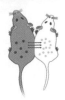

What's more serious is that those stem cells that can't survive will release a large amount of free radicals into the blood, which can cause more damage to the patient's body.

Furthermore, because stem cells survived the toxic old plasma become regulatory cells (i.e., pericytes), if the number is too large, the regulatory effects will cause confusion in the regulatory system, cancel messages released from each other, and result in lower effectiveness.

Since the main causes of death in European and American countries are acute myocardial infarctions and chronic heart failure caused by the infarction; stem cell research in Europe and the United States mostly focuses on how to apply mesenchymal stem cells to improve the function of the degraded heart. Dr. Joshua Hare of the University of Miami Professor Joshua Hare is among the one who has had the most experience.

Dr. Hare successfully isolated mesenchymal stem cells from bone marrow, and developed a storage technology that allows mesenchymal stem cells to remain stable without further differentiation during the culture process, and then established a company, i.e., Longeviron, to establish a complete mesenchymal cell bank to provide detailed HLA type-matched stem cells for clinical applications, especially for the treatment of heart disease.

Professor Hare published two important papers on the use of stem cells to treat aging frailty in 2017. His research showed that mesenchymal stem cell transplantation can exert measurable differences in patients with debilitating disease. Most patients who have received mesenchymal stem cell therapy will have more than 10% improvement in muscle strength, immunity and sexual function; this is the only double-blind controlled clinical trial result in using stem cells for the purpose of studying systemic anti-aging medicine.

The most interesting finding is that the effect of mesenchymal stem cells in the treatment of frailty is inversely related to the number of stem cells. If the experimental group is subdivided into high-dose (i.e., who received 200 Million bone marrow stem cell) and low-dose (i.e., who received 100 Million stem cells), then the clinical effect of the low-dose group will usually be better than the high-dose group in almost every measured parameters (Figure 84).

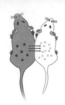

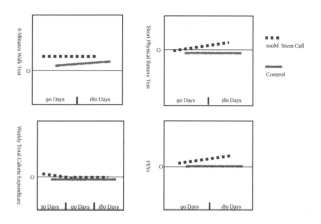

Figure 84. Experiments have found that the clinical effect of mesenchymal stem cells in the treatment of frailty is inversely related to the number of stem cells, In other words, the clinical effect of the low-dose group is much better than that of the high-dose group. (Image source: https://doi.org/10.1093/gerona/glx137)

Professor Hare's clinical trials indirectly confirmed that: although intravenous transfusion of stem cells has no direct anti-aging effect systemically, however, by secretion of cytokines it could regulate the body's immune function, and exert some systemic anti-aging effects indirectly. The role of the stem cell in Heterochronic Parabiosis treatment still could not be completely ignored. According to this, although stem cell transplantation is not a necessary step for Heterochronic Parabiosis, when Dr. Pan established the Heterochronic Parabiosis model, he decided to incorporate mesenchymal stem cell transplantation into the standard operating procedure of clinical Heterochronic Parabiosis program, and is the only optional step to be determined by the physician based on the laboratory measurement of the stem cell density and or clinical findings.

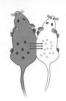

34. The 3 Steps Clinical Heterochronic Parabiosis Program.

In order to fully implement the rapid effects of conjoined Heterochronic Parabiosis on reversal of aging, Dr. Pan used the quantitative model of Heterochronic Parabiosis to calculate, and combined the two-stage Heterochronic Parabiosis treatment proposed by Dr. Kiprov with mesenchymal stem Cell transplantation therapy by Professor Hare's to introduce a three courses clinical treatment that can best simulate the conjoined Heterochronic Parabiosis.

Dr. Kiprov's two-stage Heterochronic Parabiosis treatment has several disadvantages

First, plasma exchange is expensive, and there is a 2% risk of severe complications.

Second, if FFP is used as a replacement fluid, there is a 30% rate of adverse reaction. If serum albumin and immunoglobulin are used in plasma exchange there is still a 5% rate of adverse reaction. The actual age of fresh frozen plasma donors is generally around 20 years old, which is significantly older than the adolescent plasma used in the conjoined Heterochronic

Parabiosis experiment, the clinical effect is therefore relatively limited, and risk of infection could also not be ruled out.

Third, if serum albumin and immunoglobulin are used as the replacement fluid, it cannot be replaced by the cytokines in the young plasma because most of these have a relatively short half-life.

The following detailed major concepts of the three course Heterochronic Parabiosis program designed by Dr. Pan and the reason behind the implementations based on the original hypothesis of the two-course program proposed by Dr. Kiprov.

(1) How to optimize detoxification?

The detoxification method used in the two-course Heterochronic Parabiosis is the pre-approved plasma exchange. Although it is generally regarded as safe and effective, there are still several shortcomings. First of all, when performing plasma exchange, because of the need for high-speed blood flow, it requires two large bore intravenous indwelling catchers (i.e., in and out each). However (with the exception of healthy middle-aged men) most of the patients requiring the Heterochronic Parabiosis treatment are elderly citizens. They usually have brittle veins which makes line loss quite frequent during the procedure. Furthermore, in the case of oriental female patients, their veins are relatively small, and are not likely to be able to

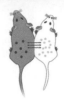

accommodate the large 18G intravenous indwelling needle required for the use of plasma exchange machines.

Secondly, because plasma exchange must pass all the human blood through a machine, the plasma proteins in a specific range of molecular weight are separated and discarded, this approach cannot completely remove all harmful proteins.

Because of the need of highly skilled technicians, human negligence is possible and may result in complications such as infection, etc...

During the plasma exchange procedure, most patients will experience a sense of panic when they see their blood exposed outside the body. With the drop in blood pressure and increase in heartbeat that frequently activates the alarming system, the process becomes quite intense both for the clients and the staff members.

When the plasma exchange procedure is performed, a dedicated technician must be nearby for counseling. The course of treatment is about 4 hours. Since the plasma exchange machine and equipment costs around 100k US dollars or more, the consumables also cost about 1,000 US dollars. Altogether, the price for each is more than $5,000.

Based on the above, traditional plasma exchange is poorly accepted by patients in non-emergency situations or in a non-hospital environment, e.g., transfusion center, anti-aging clinic, etc...

Although other detoxification therapies are also available and less expensive, most of them could only detoxify the plasma indirectly, e.g., enzyme detoxification and colon hydrotherapy detoxification. Although these processes are minimally invasive and safe, they can only exert their results in a progressive fashion, and are limited to a limited group of client-entail.

After evaluating all the detoxification methods, Dr. Pan decided to use the simplest bloodletting method which is practically of no cost; this is legitimate and is familiar to the public through campaigns of blood donation. If we follow the guideline of the blood bank regarding the volume of blood donation, for men it is limited to less than 500 ml and 250 ml for females, 6 to 10 % of toxic substances could be removed completely in each session.

In order to verify the effect of using bloodletting to eliminate toxins in the blood, Dr. Pan conducted a comparison test of plasma toxicity and activity on 150 patients before and after Heterochronic Parabiosis using the bloodletting protocol. The results showed that the toxicity of the patient's plasma could usually be improved in two to three courses of treatment, which is much more effective as compared to the improvement of

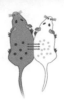

plasma activity which require usually twice or three times as many sessions.

(2) How to optimize the plasma activity?

The main proponents of the two-course Heterochronic Parabiosis are Dr. Dobri and Dr. Conboy. They are both based in the Bay Area of California, USA. They use serum albumin and immunoglobulin from plasma manufacturers. Since serum albumin and immunoglobulin are quite expensive protein components, if high concentrations of albumin and globulin are used, the cost of treatment will be high.

According to the analysis of proteome study of young and old plasma by Wyss-Coray, there are only a few types of proteins that are unique to the young plasma. Dr. Pan used the adolescent plasma collected in Phnom Penh to perform limited analysis and compare with the proteome data of Wyss-Coray, and developed a formulation using protein drugs that are commercially available in the market, to simulate the natural adolescent plasma.

In order to better mimic the concentration of beneficial factors in the plasma, Dr. Pan further separated the short-acting protein from the long-acting proteins, and allowed them to be injected in intervals based on detailed calculation of the half-lives of each component.

(3) How to optimize Stem cell transplantation?

Since the patients receiving the Heterochronic Parabiosis treatment are over 50 years old, the quality of the client's own stem cells is obviously insufficient compared with the stem cells of young people or newborn babies. In order to achieve the best effect, after multiple evaluations, since most of the countries have public cord blood banks and provide affordable and certified cord stem cells, Dr. Pan decided to use mesenchymal stem cells from the government cord blood banks as the source of stem cells for the HP program.

Before transplantation, the plasma toxicity and activity of the client should be examined. If the plasma toxicity is high, the survival rate of the implanted umbilical cord stem cells will be very low, which is equivalent to discarding the precious stem cells. If the activity of the plasma is low, the stem cells mounted in the lungs will quickly enter a state of hibernation, will not be able to produce cytokines in accordance with the state of the patient's conditions, and the clinical effect will be sub-optimal.

Based on the results of Professor Hare's experiments, Dr. Pan uses progressive stem cell transplantation, that is to transplant a small amount of mesenchymal stem cells each time after the toxicity and activity of the plasma become viable to the stem cell to be transplanted, evaluate the effects two weeks later, and adjust the numbers accordingly. In this way, not only the clinical

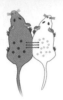

effect is improved; the number of stem cells and the cost are also greatly reduced by as much as 80%.

The three-course therapy can also be used in conjunction with the two-course therapy. For business people who want to maintain their vitality, muscle strength and improve their sub-health state, they will only require three-course treatment annually and two-course therapy on a quarter or semi-annually basis.

As for patients who have moderate to severe disease conditions, they will need to have a full physical examination, laboratory tests, and plasma toxicity and activity test, and plan the treatment program based on the evaluation of the physician.

35. Really? Trilogy Of Scientific Breakthrough

All technology development usually goes through the four stages of business development, that are Discovery, Development, Promotion, and Commercialization. All major advances in the sciences also go through the following three stages.

Professor Takeshi Oka of the Department of Chemistry at the University of Chicago stated clearly at the end of his Keynote Address on "A life with one molecule H3+: Astronomy and Chemistry" about his remarkable discovery of interstellar H3+ in the molecular clouds at the Academic Sinica on Mar. 7, 2019: "When I was attempting it, people said it was impossible. When I found it, people was skeptical. When it was all established and the dust was settled people said it was obvious. "

Let us look into the insights of his statement. The first stage is Impossible: Because what a scientist with a big vision sees cannot be understood by most people, when Dr. Carrel and Dr. Kiprov proposed the concept of clinical Heterochronic Parabiosis, most people sneered at the concept of clinical Heterochronic Parabiosis, thinking it was impossible.

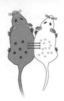

The second stage is skeptical and peer slander. When new technologies are launched on the market, in order to survive, they must start charging a fee. Therefore, many scientists will be considered to be deceiving for personal gain by the public. Coupled with the inevitable defensiveness of those with vested interests and the mentality of literati disdain, malicious attacks by peers behind the back have become the norm.

The third stage is the acceptance stage. At this stage, after the publication of more and more papers, the endorsements of users, and media exposures, new scientific discoveries will be made familiar to the public. Knowing that it will be regarded as not keeping up with the times, professionals working in related industries are forced to switch from a confrontational standpoint to investing and accepting new technologies in order to maintain customer relationships which are the source of their income.

After 100 years of development, the treatment of Heterochronic Parabiosis experienced by at least tens of thousands of people, to this day is still in its very early stage, so it will be questioned and challenged by most physicians and scientists.

36. Pregnancy Is Heterochronic Parabiosis

Other than the conjoined, intravenous, and transdermal heterochronic parabiosis discussed previously there are still other types of heterochronic parabiosis. Notably, pregnancy of mammals is actually a Heterochronic Parabiosis in a natural way. Different from Dr. Carrel's experiment, where the coupling is approximately equal in size and weight; the size of the old-young pair in pregnancy are quite different. (Figure 85) Therefore, pregnancy could be regarded as an asymmetric conjoined Heterochronic Parabiosis.

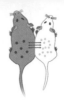

FETUS IN UTERO
PREGNANCY WOMAN DIAGRAMS

Placenta

Umbilical cord

Uterus

Abdominal
muscle wall

Urinary bladder

Pubic symphysis

Urethra

Cervix

Vagina

Rectum

Anus

Figure 85. Pregnancy is a Heterochronic Parabiosis asymmetrical in size.
(Image source: freepik.com)

In order to compare the effect of different kinds of parabiosis, Dr. Pan set up an index called HPI (Heterochronic Parabiosis Index). He defined this index as the weight ratio x conjoined time. For example, the average weight of the fetus in the last three months is about 3 kg, and the mother's weight is about 60 kg. Therefore, the size of the fetus is only one-twentieth that of the mother. As for the conjoined time, because the fetal size is also negligent in the first and second trimester, therefore, only the third trimester is calculated, which is about 90 days. Multiplying 0.05 by 90, we can then calculate the Heterochronic Parabiosis index as 4.5. As for the size ratio of Dr. Carrel's conjoined Heterochronic Parabiosis is approximately 1.0, and the conjoined time is about ten days, after we multiply these two numbers, we can calculate the Heterochronic Parabiosis index to be 10.0, so that the clinical rejuvenation effect of pregnancy on the mother's physical function is equivalent to 50% of the surgical conjoined Heterochronic Parabiosis. (Figure 86)

Rejuvenating effect of pregnancy on the mother

Tal Falick Michaeli, M.D.,[a] Yehudit Bergman, Ph.D.,[a] and Yuval Gielchinsky, M.D., Ph.D.[a,b]

[a] Rubin Chair in Medical Science, Department of Developmental Biology and Cancer Research, IMRIC, Hebrew University-Hadassah Medical School; and [b] Department of Obstetrics and Gynecology, Hadassah-Hebrew University Medical Center, Jerusalem, Israel

Aging is associated with reduced tissue regenerative capacity. In recent years, studies in mice have shown that transfusion of blood from young animals to old ones can reverse some aging effects and increase regenerative potential similar to that seen in young animals. Because pregnancy is a unique biological model of a partially shared blood system, we have speculated that pregnancy would have a rejuvenating effect on the mother. Recent studies support this idea. In this review, we will summarize the current knowledge of the rejuvenating effect of pregnancy on the mother. (Fertil Steril® 2015;103:1125–8. ©2015 by American Society for Reproductive Medicine.)
Key Words: Aging, regeneration, rejuvenation, pregnancy

Discuss: You can discuss this article with its authors and with other ASRM members at http://fertstertforum.com/michaelit-rejuvenation-pregnancy-mother/

Use your smartphone to scan this QR code and connect to the discussion forum for this article now.*

* Download a free QR code scanner by searching for "QR scanner" in your smartphone's app store or app marketplace.

Figure 86 Pregnancy has an anti-aging and rejuvenating effect on the mother. (Source: fertstert.org)

Tal Michaeli, Yehudit Bergman and Yuval Gielchinsky of Hebrew University in Israel, used anthropologic data to explore

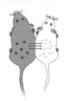

the rejuvenation benefits of pregnancy on mother. They compared the effects of pregnancy on the mother's life expectancy based on demographic data. They took two groups of mothers (i.e., the total number of child bearing in the two groups was basically the same), from the government record. The first group of mothers gave birth to their last child at age of 45, and the second group of mothers gave birth to their last child at age of 35. Because the time of effective circulatory connection of the mother-child is 90 days, it is assumed that the blood of the mother and the blood of the fetus can be mixed completely.

Although the ages of the mothers in the two groups are different, the age of the fetus is roughly 1 year old (correctly speaking, it should be 6 to 9 months). Because the gap between 45-year-old and 0-year-old is relatively large, it is reasonable to speculate that the 45-year-old pregnancy will have a better rejuvenation effect than the 35-year-old pregnancy on the mother.

The results of this population lifespan study showed that a mother who was 45 years old at the time of her last pregnancy was more likely to live to 80 years of age as compared to a mother who was 35 years old at the time of her last pregnancy by a large 50% margin (Figure 87). This study is considered to be a Level 3 clinical trial for the effect of Heterochronic Parabiosis on rejuvenation and lifespan extension. It is enough to become a treatment guideline for anti aging physicians who are interested in the practice of anti-aging medicine based on the Principle of Heterochronic Parabiosis.

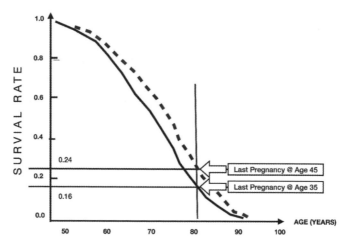

Figure 87. The results of the study of expectancy show that the women who gave last birth at age of 45, is 50% more likely to live to the age of 80 as compared to women who gave birth to their last child at age of 35. This study is considered to be the ultimate evidence that Heterochronic Parabiosis can reverse aging and prolong life.

Generally speaking, the average life expectancy of women around the world is about 10% longer than that of men. From adolescence to the beginning of menopause, women must undergo detoxification by menstruation every month. Furthermore, most of them will have the benefit of the

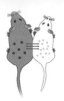

rejuvenation effect of pregnancy from conjoined Heterochronic Parabiosis with their fetus. This incidentally provides the answer to the reason why women live longer than men in the world.

Heterochronic Parabiosis
Anti-aging Plasma Exchange

37. The Future Of Heterochronic Parabiosis Technologies

Heterochronic Parabiosis is currently the only method that can reverse aging rapidly. It can improve the memory and cognitive function of the central nervous system. It could reduce chronic inflammation and insulin resistance, therefore, might assist in management of T2DM. Furthermore, it could also improve kidney function, and reduce the risk of recurrence and metastasis of cancer.

Clinically, there are many ways to accomplish the results of Heterochronic Parabiosis. The most natural way is to get pregnant. By sharing the blood of the fetus during pregnancy, organs of the mother can benefit from the effect of aging reversal. The older the mother is, the clearer the effect. Unfortunately, the baby must also pay the same price, which potentially leads to more health problems after birth as the age of mother increases or conditions worsen.

The use of surgery to allow two animals, young and old, to share the blood circulatory system, thereby reversing the function of aging organs, was first performed by Dr. Carrel of the University of Chicago who is also the Nobel laureate in 1912. This method

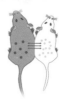

is also the most thoroughly studied method, but unfortunately it is almost impossible to implement in clinical practice.

For 100 years, scientists and doctors all over the world have wanted to apply Dr. Carrel's conjoined Heterochronic Parabiosis method to reverse the function of aging organs in humans, but the progress is very limited.

There are finally several clinically feasible solutions in the early 21st century. Not only have all of them entered the clinic, they have also become more and more accepted in the market.

The mutual complementation of Yin and Yang, proposed by Chinese Taoism thousands of years ago, is also a kind of Heterochronic Parabiosis. Although this method of exchanging body fluids through the mucous membranes of male and female sexual organs has a long history, it is limited by the efficacy of absorption just like its transdermal counterpart. The systemic anti-aging effect of the cytokines exchanged through mucosa still needs to be verified by future experiments and clinical trials.

There are many other types of plasma therapy used in the treatment of Heterochronic Parabiosis in the medical field. For example, the serum of patients with new Covid-19 is used as the source of antibodies for patients with severe diseases (i.e., convalescent plasma therapy), or the use of athletes' Plasma to increase metabolism (i.e., exercise plasma weight loss therapy) and so on.

These science and technology companies, which look like a fantasy, have received a lot of venture capital funding in recent years. Related treatments have also entered the first and second phases of clinical trials in Europe, America, and Japan. Future development should be just around the corner.

Finally, beginning 2019, some university laboratories and biotech companies have begun to study the use of in vitro Heterochronic Parabiosis to reverse the function of aging organs. These technologies were originally used to improve the yield of donor organs during organ transplantation. It is hoped that in the near future, they can replace the needs of traditional organ transplantation and greatly improve human health and well-being!

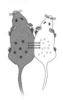

38. References

Abdul Halim Abdul Jalil. (2017) Hope For Untreatable Medical Disorders with Live Cell Therapy. Matador Press. ASIN: B072JYS36H

Advances in Recombinant Human Growth Hormone Replacement Therapy in Adults. https://pituitary.mgh.harvard.edu/ef-944.htm. Neuroendocrine and Pituitary Tumor Clinical Center, Harvard Medical School

Ahmed, AS, Sheng, MH, Wasnik, S., Baylink, DJ, & Lau, KW (2017). Effect of aging on stem cells. World Journal of Experimental Medicine, 7(1), 1–10. https://doi.org/10.5493/wjem.v7.i1.1

Akhtar A. (2015). The flaws and human harms of animal experimentation. Cambridge quarterly of healthcare ethics: CQ: the international journal of healthcare ethics committees, 24(4), 407–419. https://doi.org/10.1017/S0963180115000079

Belikov AV (2019). Age-related diseases are vicious cycles. Ageing research reviews, 49, 11–26. https://doi.org/10.1016/j.arr.2018.11.002

Benveniste GL (2013). Alexis Carrel: the good, the bad, the ugly. ANZ journal of surgery, 83(9), 609–611. https://doi.org/10.1111/ans.12167

Bhattacharjee, RN. (2019) Subnormothermic Oxygenated Perfusion Optimally Preserves Donor Kidneys Ex Vivo Published: May 21, 2019 DOI: https://doi.org/10.1016/j.ekir.2019.05.013

Bianconi, E., Piovesan, A., Facchin, F., Beraudi, A., Casadei, R., Frabetti, F., Vitale, L., Pelleri, MC, Tassani, S., Piva, F., Perez - Amodio, S., Strippoli, P., & Canaider, S. (2013). An estimation of the number of cells in the human body. Annals of human biology, 40(6), 463–471

Block, TJ, Marinkovic, M., Tran, ON, Gonzalez, AO, Marshall, A., Dean, DD, & Chen, XD (2017). Restoring the quantity and quality of elderly human mesenchymal stem cells for autologous cell-based therapies. Stem cell research & therapy, 8(1), 239. https://doi.org/10.1186/s13287-017-0688-x

Boada, M., López, O., Núñez, L., Szczepiorkowski, ZM, Torres, M., Grifols, C., & Páez, A. (2019). Plasma exchange for Alzheimer's disease Management by Albumin Replacement

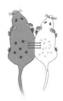

(AMBAR) trial: Study design and progress. Alzheimer's & dementia (New York, NY), 5, 61–69. https://doi.org/10.1016/j.trci.2019.01.001

Burt, RK, & Marmont, AM, (2004) Stem Cell Therapy and Auto-immune Diseases, CRC Press, ISBN-13: 978-1587060311

Caplan, Arnold. (2017)'The science behind adipose derived MSCs and their potential applications, Orthopaedics at the ROCKSTAR Kongress, London. https://www.youtube.com/watch?v=A4fX88LRuCg

Caplan, A. (2017) Mesenchymal Stem Cells: Time to Change the Name! Stem Cell Translational Medicine 6:1445–1451, https://doi.org/10.1002/sctm.17-0051

Carrel, A. (1912) Suture of Blood-Vessels and Transplantation of Organs, Nobel Lecture, https://www.nobelprize.org/prizes/medicine/1912/carrel/lecture/

Castellano JM (2019). Blood-Based Therapies to Combat Aging. Gerontology, 65(1), 84-89. https://doi.org/10.1159/000492573

Chaisinthop N., (2013) What is Fresh Cell Therapy, Center For Bionetworking.

http://www.centreforbionetworking.org/wp-content/uploads/2013/12/What-is-Fresh-Cell-Therapy.pdf

Choi EW (2009). Adult stem cell therapy for autoimmune disease. International journal of stem cells, 2(2), 122–128. https://doi.org/10.15283/ijsc.2009.2.2.122

Colangelo, D., Robbins, P., Nasto, LA, Niedemhofer,, L., Pola, E.. (2016) Heterochronic Parabiosis Approach: is it Possible to Interrupt the Aging Process of the Intervertebral Disc Degeneration? An in vivo Experimental Study. Global Spine Journal DOI: 10.1055/s-0036-1582615

Conboy, IM, Conboy, MJ, Wagers, AJ, Girma, ER, Weissman, IL, & Rando, TA (2005). Rejuvenation of aged progenitor cells by exposure to a young systemic environment. Nature, 433(7027), 760– 764. https://doi.org/10.1038/nature03260
Conboy, IM, & Rando, TA (2012). Heterochronic parabiosis for the study of the effects of aging on stem cells and their niches. Cell cycle (Georgetown, Tex.), 11(12), 2260–2267. https:/ /doi.org/10.4161/cc.20437

Conboy, MJ, Conboy, IM, & Rando, TA (2013). Heterochronic parabiosis: historical perspective and methodological considerations for studies of aging and longevity. Aging cell, 12(3), 525–530. https://doi.org /10.1111/acel.12065

Conese, M., Carbone, A., Beccia, E., & Angiolillo, A. (2017). The Fountain of Youth: A Tale of Parabiosis, Stem Cells, and Rejuvenation. Open medicine (Warsaw, Poland), 12, 376–383. https://doi.org/10.1515/med-2017-0053

Corbyn, Z. (2020) Could young blood stop us getting old? https://www.theguardian.com/society/2020/feb/02/could-young-blood-stop-us-getting-old-transfusions-experiments - mice-plasma, The Guardian

Cox, D. (2019) The new growth in hair loss research. The Guardian. https://www.theguardian.com/lifeandstyle/2019/sep/07/new-hair-loss-research-balding-medical-treatments

Cunningham, CJ, Redondo-Castro, E., & Allan, SM (2018). The therapeutic potential of the mesenchymal stem cell secretome in ischaemic stroke. Journal of cerebral blood flow and metabolism: official journal of the International Society of Cerebral Blood Flow and Metabolism, 38(8), 1276–1292. https://doi.org/10.1177/0271678X18776802

D e Cabo, R., & Mattson, MP (2019). Effects of Intermittent Fasting on Health, Aging, and Disease. The New England Journal of medicine, 381(26), 2541–2551. https://doi.org /10.1056/NEJMra1905136

De Witte, S., Merino, AM, Franquesa, M., Strini, T., van Zoggel, J., Korevaar, SS, Luk, F., Gargesha, M., O'Flynn, L., Roy, D., Elliman, SJ, Newsome, PN, Baan, CC, & Hoogduijn, MJ (2017). Cytokine treatment optimises the immunotherapeutic effects of umbilical cord-derived MSC for treatment of inflammatory liver disease. Stem cell research & therapy, 8(1), 140. https://doi.org/10.1186/s13287-017-0590-6

Díez, JJ, Sangiao-Alvarellos, S., & Cordido, F. (2018). Treatment with Growth Hormone for Adults with Growth Hormone Deficiency Syndrome: Benefits and Risks. International journal of molecular sciences, 19(3), 893. https ://doi.org/10.3390/ijms19030893

Dinh, PC, Paudel, D., Brochu, H., Popowski, KD, Gracieux, MC, Cores, J., Huang, K., Hensley, MT, Harrell, E., Vandergriff, AC, George, AK, Barrio , RT, Hu, S., Allen, TA, Blackburn, K., Caranasos, TG, Peng, X., Schnabel, LV, Adler, KB, Doidge, N., (2015) The Brain's Way of Healing, Viking Penguin

Dufner-Almeida, LG, Cruz, D., Mingroni Netto, RC, Batissoco, AC, Oiticica, J., & Salazar-Silva, R. (2019). Stem-cell therapy for hearing loss: are we there yet? Brazilian journal of otorhinolaryngology, 85(4), 520–529. https://doi.org/10.1016/j.bjorl.2019.04.006

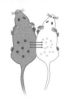

Epifanova, MV, Gvasalia, BR, Durashov, MA, Artenmenko, SA. (2020) Platelet-Rich Plasma Therapy for Male Sexual Dysfunction: Myth or Reality? Sex Med Rev 8:106-113., https://doi.org /10.1016/j.sxmr.2019.02.002

Falick Michaeli, T., Bergman, Y., & Gielchinsky, Y. (2015). Rejuvenating effect of pregnancy on the mother. Fertility and sterility, 103(5), 1125–1128. https://doi.org/10.1016 /j.fertnstert.2015.02.034

Franceschi, C., Garagnani, P., Morsiani, C., Conte, M., Santoro, A., Grignolio, A., Monti, D., Capri, M., & Salvioli, S. (2018). The Continuum of Aging and Age-Related Diseases: Common Mechanisms but Different Rates. Frontiers in medicine, 5, 61. https://doi.org/10.3389/fmed.2018.00061

Gentile, P., Cole, JP, Cole, MA, Garcovich, S., Bielli, A., Scioli, MG, Orlandi, A., Insalaco, C., & Cervelli, V. (2017). Evaluation of Not- Activated and Activated PRP in Hair Loss Treatment: Role of Growth Factor and Cytokine Concentrations Obtained by Different Collection Systems. International journal of molecular sciences, 18(2), 408. https://doi.org/10.3390/ijms18020408

Gentile, P., Garcovich, S., Bielli, A., Scioli, MG, Orlandi, A., & Cervelli, V. (2015). The Effect of Platelet-Rich Plasma in Hair

Regrowth: A Randomized Placebo-Controlled Trial . Stem cells translational medicine, 4(11), 1317–1323. https://doi.org/10.5966/sctm.2015-0107

Golpanian, S., DiFede, DL, Khan, A., Schulman, IH, Landin, AM, Tompkins, BA, Heldman, AW, Miki, R., Goldstein, BJ, Mushtaq, M., Levis-Dusseau, S. , Byrnes, JJ, Lowery, M., Natsumeda, M., Delgado, C., Saltzman, R., Vidro-Casiano, M., Pujol, MV, Da Fonseca, M., Oliva, AA, Jr,... Hare , JM (2017). Allogeneic Human Mesenchymal Stem Cell Infusions for Aging Frailty. The journals of gerontology. Series A, Biological sciences and medical sciences, 72(11), 1505–1512. https://doi.org/10.1093/gerona /glx056

Gonzalez-Armenta, JL, Mahapatra, G., Allison Amick, K., Li, N., Lu, B., & Molina, A. (2018). Heterochronic Parabiosis: Old Blood Attenuates Mitochondrial Bioenergetics of Young Mice. Innovation in Aging, 2 (Suppl 1), 558. https://doi.org/10.1093/geroni/igy023.2064

Gowen, A., Shahjin, F., Chand, S., Odegaard, KE, & Yelamanchili, SV (2020). Mesenchymal Stem Cell-Derived Extracellular Vesicles: Challenges in Clinical Applications. Frontiers in cell and developmental biology, 8, 149 . https://doi.org/10.3389/fcell.2020.00149

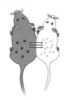

Guenthart, BA, O'Neill, JD, Kim, J., Queen, D., Chicotka, S., Fung, K., Simpson, M., Donocoff, R., Salna, M., Marboe, CC, Cunningham , K., Halligan, SP, Wobma, HM, Hozain, AE, Romanov, A., Vunjak-Novakovic, G., & Bacchetta, M. (2019). Regeneration of severely damaged lungs using an interventional cross-circulation platform. Nature communications, 10(1), 1985. https://doi.org/10.1038/s41467-019-09908-1

Hans-Georg Müller, Jeng-Min Chiou, James R. Carey, Jane-Ling Wang, Fertility and Life Span: Late Children Enhance Female Longevity, The Journals of Gerontology: Series A, Volume 57, Issue 5, 1 May 2002, Pages B202–B206, https://doi.org/10.1093/gerona/57.5.B202

Hansen, M., Rubinsztein, DC & Walker, DW Autophagy as a promoter of longevity: insights from model organisms. Nat Rev Mol Cell Biol 19, 579–593 (2018). https://doi.org/10.1038/s41580- 018-0033-y Harding, A.. (2014) More compounds failing phase I. The Scientist. https://www.the-scientist.com/news-analysis/more-compounds-failing-phase-i-49707

Hare, J.. (2011) Clinical Research Protocol :A Phase I/II, Randomized Pilot Study of the Comparative Safety and Efficacy of Trans-endocardial Injection of Autologous Mesenchymal Stem Cells Versus Allogeneic Mesenchymal Stem Cells in

Patients With Chronic Ischemic Left Ventricular Dysfunction Secondary to Myocardial Infarction.

Hare, JM, DiFede, DL, Rieger, AC, Florea, V., Landin, AM, El-Khorazaty, J., Khan, A., Mushtaq, M., Lowery, MH, Byrnes, JJ, Hendel, RC, Cohen, MG, Alfonso, CE, Valasaki, K., Pujol, MV, Golpanian, S., Ghersin, E., Fishman, JE, Pattany, P., Gomes, SA, Heldman, AW (2017). Randomized Comparison of Allogeneic Versus Autologous Mesenchymal Stem Cells for Nonischemic Dilated Cardiomyopathy: POSEIDON-DCM Trial. Journal of the American College of Cardiology, 69(5), 526–537. https://doi.org/10.1016/j.jacc.2016.11.009

Harris, JP (2018) Regenerating Hair Cells to Treat Hearing Loss, https://www.youtube.com/watch?v=cZd-Rg-7xzE

Haney, NM, Gabrielson, A., Kohn, TP, & Hellstrom, W. (2019). The Use of Stromal Vascular Fraction in the Treatment of Male Sexual Dysfunction: A Review of Preclinical and Clinical Studies. Sexual medicine reviews, 7(2), 313–320. https://doi.org/10.1016/j.sxmr.2018.04.001

Hass, R., Kasper, C., Böhm, S., & Jacobs, R. (2011). Different populations and sources of human mesenchymal stem cells (MSC): A comparison of adult and neonatal tissue-derived MSC. Cell communication and signaling: CCS, 9, 12. https://doi.org/10.1186/1478-811X-9-12

Heron, M. (2017) Deaths: Leading Causes for 2017. National Vital Statistics Reports 68, 6.
https://www.cdc.gov/nchs/data/nvsr/nvsr68/nvsr68_06-508.pdf

Hong, P., Yang, H., Wu, Y., Li, K., & Tang, Z. (2019). The functions and clinical application potential of exosomes derived from adipose mesenchymal stem cells: a comprehensive review. Stem cell research & therapy, 10(1), 242.
https://doi.org/10.1186/s13287-019-1358-y

Horwitz, EM, Prockop, DJ, Fitzpatrick, LA, Koo, WW, Gordon, PL, Neel, M., Sussman, M., Orchard, P., Marx, JC, Pyeritz, RE, & Brenner, MK (1999) . Transplantability and therapeutic effects of bone marrow-derived mesenchymal cells in children with osteogenesis imperfecta. Nature medicine, 5(3), 309-313.
https://doi.org/10.1038/6529

Horwitz, EM, & Dominici, M. (2008). How do mesenchymal stromal cells exert their therapeutic benefit?. Cytotherapy, 10(8), 771-774. https://doi.org/10.1080/14653240802618085

Kadry, MH (2018) Autologous Adipose Derived Stem Cell versus Platelet Rich Plasma Injection in the Treatment of Androgenetic Alopecia: Efficacy, Side Effects and Safety. J Clin. Exp. Dermatol. Res. 9:3

Kassis, I., Zangi, L., Rivkin, R., Levdansky, L., Samuel, S., Marx, G., & Gorodetsky, R. (2006). Isolation of mesenchymal stem cells from G-CSF-mobilized human peripheral blood using fibrin microbeads. Bone marrow transplantation, 37(10), 967–976. https://doi.org/10.1038/sj.bmt.1705358

Kieb, M., Sander, F., Prinz, C., Adam, S., Mau-Möller, A., Bader, R., Peters, K., & Tischer, T. (2017). Platelet-Rich Plasma Powder: A New Preparation Method for the Standardization of Growth Factor Concentrations. The American journal of sports medicine, 45(4), 954–960. https://doi.org/10.1177/0363546516674475

Kim, HO, Kim, HS, Youn, JC, Shin, EC, & Park, S. (2011). Serum cytokine profiles in healthy young and elderly population assessed using multiplexed bead-based immunoassays. Journal of translational medicine, 9, 113 . https://doi.org/10.1186/1479-5876-9-113

Kiprov D. (2013). Intermittent heterochronic plasma exchange as a modality for delaying cellular senescence-a hypothesis. Journal of clinical apheresis, 28(6), 387–389. https://doi.org/10.1002/jca.21286

Lee, RC, River, LP, Pan, FS, Ji, L., & Wollmann, RL (1992). Surfactant-induced sealing of electropermeabilized skeletal muscle membranes in vivo. Proceedings of the National

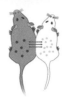

Academy of Sciences of the United States of America , 89(10), 4524–4528. https://doi.org/10.1073/pnas.89.10.4524

Lehallier, B., Gate, D., Schaum, N., Nanasi, T., Lee, SE, Yousef, H., Moran Losada, P., Berdnik, D., Keller, A., Verghese, J., Sathyan, S., Franceschi, C., Milman, S., Barzilai, N., & Wyss-Coray, T. (2019). Undulating changes in human plasma proteome profiles across the lifespan. Nature medicine, 25(12), 1843–1850. https://doi.org/10.1038/s41591-019-0673-2

Leibacher, J., & Henschler, R. (2016). Biodistribution, migration and homing of systemically applied mesenchymal stem/stromal cells. Stem cell research & therapy, 7, 7.
https://doi.org/10.1186/s13287- 015-0271-2

Liu, STH, Lin, H., Baine, I. et al. (2020) Convalescent plasma treatment of severe COVID-19: a propensity score–matched control study. Nat Med. Https://doi.org/10.1038/s41591 -020-1088-9

Loffredo, FS, Steinhauser, ML, Jay, SM, Gannon, J., Pancoast, JR, Yalamanchi, P., Sinha, M., Dall'Osso, C., Khong, D., Shadrach, JL, Miller, CM , Singer, BS, Stewart, A., Psychogios, N., Gerszten, RE, Hartigan, AJ, Kim, MJ, Serwold, T., Wagers, AJ, & Lee, RT (2013). Growth differentiation factor 11 is a circulating factor that reverses age-related cardiac hypertrophy. Cell, 153(4), 828–839.

https://doi.org/10.1016/j.cell.2013.04.015

Lobo, LJ, Cheng, K. (2020). Inhalation of lung spheroid cell secretome and exosomes promotes lung repair in pulmonary fibrosis. Nature communications, 11(1), 1064. https://doi.org/10.1038/s41467-020 -14344-7

Mahmoudi, S., Xu, L., & Brunet, A. (2019). Turning back time with emerging rejuvenation strategies. Nature cell biology, 21(1), 32–43. https://doi.org/10.1038/ s41556-018-0206-0

Malchesky PS (2018). Aging, Disease, and Therapeutic Apheresis. Therapeutic Apheresis and Dialysis: Official Peer-Review Journal of the International Society for Apheresis, the Japanese Society for Apheresis, the Japanese Society for Dialysis Therapy, 22(4), 312 -316. https://doi.org/10.1111/1744-9987.12706

Manzelou J. (2016) Menopause Reversal Restore Periods and produces fertile eggs. https://www.newscientist.com/article/mg23130833-100-menopause-reversal-restores-periods-and-produces-fertile-eggs/, New Scientist .

Marshak, DR, Gardner, RL, D. Gottlieb. (2001) Stem Cell Biology. Cold Spring Harbor Laboratory Press.

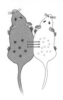

Maxmen A., (2017) Questionable "Young Blood" Transfusions Offered in US as Anti-Aging Remedy. https://www.technologyreview.com/s/603242/questionable-young-blood-transfusions-offered-in-us-   as-anti-aging-remedy/. MIT Technology Review.

Medina, MA, 3rd, Nguyen, JT, Kirkham, JC, Lee, JH, McCormack, MC, Randolph, MA, & Austen, WG, Jr (2011). Polymer therapy: a novel treatment to improve fat graft viability.Plastic and reconstructive surgery, 127(6), 2270–2282. https://doi.org/10.1097/PRS.0b013e3182139fc1

Middeldorp, J., Lehallier, B., Villeda, SA, Miedema, SS, Evans, E., Czirr, E., Zhang, H., Luo, J., Stan, T., Mosher, KI, Masliah, E ., & Wyss-Coray, T. (2016). Preclinical Assessment of Young Blood Plasma for Alzheimer Disease. JAMA neurology, 73(11), 1325–1333. https://doi.org/10.1001/jamaneurol.2016.3185

Milo, R., Phillips, R.. (2015) Cell Biology by the numbers. Garland Science.

Miyamoto, H., Nosé, Y.. (2010) Can an Apheresis Therapy become an Effective Method for Anti-aging Medicine? Anti-Aging Medicine 7 (9): 100–106. https://www.jstage.jst.go.jp/article/jaam/7/9/7_9_100/_article

Murphy, M., Moncivais, K. & Caplan, A. Mesenchymal stem cells: environmentally responsive therapeutics for regenerative medicine. Exp Mol Med 45, e54 (2013). https://doi.org/10.1038/emm.2013.94

Nakayama S, Kodama K, Oguchi K. (1989) [A comparative study of human placenta hydrolysate (Laennec) by intravenous or subcutaneous injection on liver regeneration after partial hepatectomy in normal and CCl4-induced cirrhosis rats]. Nihon Yakurigaku Zasshi. Nov; 94(5):289-97. Japanese. doi: 10.1254/fpj.94.289. PMID: 2613108

Narbonne P. (2018). The effect of age on stem cell function and utility for therapy. Cell medicine, 10, 2155179018773756. https://doi.org/10.1177/2155179018773756

Oliva, AA, McClain-Moss, L, Pena, A, Drouillard, A, Hare, JM. Allogeneic mesenchymal stem cell therapy: A regenerative medicine approach to geroscience. Aging Med. 2019; 2: 142–146. https:// doi.org/10.1002/agm2.12079

Ouryazdanpanah, N., Dabiri, S., Derakhshani, A., Vahidi, R., & Farsinejad, A. (2018). Peripheral Blood-Derived Mesenchymal Stem Cells: Growth Factor-Free Isolation, Molecular Characterization and Differentiation. Iranian journal of pathology, 13(4), 461-466

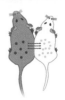

Palm, W., Park, Y., Wright, K., Pavlova, NN, Tuveson, DΛ, & Thompson, CB (2015). The Utilization of Extracellular Proteins as Nutrients Is Suppressed by mTORC1. Cell, 162(2), 259–270. https://doi.org/10.1016/j.cell.2015.06.017

Pan, FS, Stephen Chen; Robert A. Mintzer; Chin-Tu Chen; Paul Schumacker (1990) Studies of yeast cell oxygenation and energetics by laser fluorometry of reduced nicotinamide adenine dinucleotide. SPIE Proceedings Vol. 1396: Applications of Optical Engineering: Proceedings of OE/Midwest '90 Rudolph P. Guzik; Hans E. Eppinger; Richard E. Gillespie; Mary Kathryn Dubiel; James E. Pearson, Editor(s)

Pan, FS (2019) Fountain of Youth, University of Chicago Alumni Event. https://www.uchicago.cn/events/alumni-event-fountain-of-youth/

Pan, FS (2020) Advances in Facial Rejuvenation Technologies. Keynote, Annual Conference, International Federation of Facial Plastic Surgery Societies. https://www.iffpss2020.org/Speaker

Peggy A. Lockhart, Peter Martin, Mary Ann Johnson, Elizabeth Shirtcliff, Leonard W. Poon, The Relationship of Fertility, Lifestyle, and Longevity Among Women, The Journals of Gerontology: Series A, Volume 72, Issue 6, 1 June 2017, Pages 754–759, https://doi.org/10.1093/gerona/glw158

Phinney, DG, & Pittenger, MF (2017). Concise Review: MSC-Derived Exosomes for Cell-Free Therapy. Stem cells (Dayton, Ohio), 35(4), 851–858. https://doi.org/ 10.1002/stem.2575

Pittenger, MF, Discher, DE, Péault, BM, Phinney, DG, Hare, JM, & Caplan, AI (2019). Mesenchymal stem cell perspective: cell biology to clinical progress. NPJ Regenerative medicine, 4, 22. https://doi.org/10.1038/s41536-019-0083-6

Powell K. (2009). Irina Conboy: making the old feel young again. Interview by Kendall Powell. The Journal of cell biology, 187(1), 4–5. https://doi.org/10.1083/jcb.1871pi

Rando TA (2006). Stem cells, ageing and the quest for immortality. Nature, 441(7097), 1080–1086. https://doi.org/10.1038/nature04958

Rea, IM, Gibson, DS, McGilligan, V., McNerlan, SE, Alexander, HD, & Ross, OA (2018). Age and Age-Related Diseases: Role of Inflammation Triggers and Cytokines. Frontiers in immunology, 9, 586 . https://doi.org/10.3389/fimmu.2018.00586

Rebo, J., Mehdipour, M., Gathwala, R., Causey, K., Liu, Y., Conboy reveal, MJ, & Conboy, IM (2016). A single

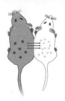

heterochronic blood exchanges rapid inhibition of multiple tissues by old blood. Nature communications, 7, 13363. https://doi.org/10.1038/ncomms13363

Reedy, Brian KMD; Pan, Fushih MD, Ph.D.; Kim, Won Seok MD; Gannon, Francis HMD; Krasinskas, Alyssa MD; Bartlett, Scott PMD Properties of Coralline Hydroxyapatite and Expanded Polytetrafluoroethylene Membrane in the Immature Craniofacial Skeleton, Plastic and Reconstructive Surgery: January 1999-Volume 103-Issue 1-p 20-26

Reedy, Brian KMD; Pan, Fushih MD, Ph.D.; Kim, Won Seok MD; Bartlett, Scott PMD The Direct Effect of Intraorbital Pressure on Orbital Growth in the Anophthalmic Piglet, Plastic and Reconstructive Surgery: September 1999-Volume 104- Issue 3-p 713-718

Rudman, D., Feller, AG, Nagraj, HS, Gergans, GA, Lalitha, PY, Goldberg, AF, Schlenker, RA, Cohn, L., Rudman, IW, & Mattson, DE (1990). Effects of human growth hormone in men over 60 years old. The New England journal of medicine, 323(1), 1–6. https://doi.org/10.1056/NEJM199007053230101

Schulman, IH, Balkan, W., & Hare, JM (2018). Mesenchymal Stem Cell Therapy for Aging Frailty. Frontiers in nutrition, 5, 108. https://doi.org/10.3389/fnut.2018.00108

Scott, S., Roberts, M., & Chung, E. (2019). Platelet-Rich Plasma and Treatment of Erectile Dysfunction: Critical Review of Literature and Global Trends in Platelet-Rich Plasma Clinics. Sexual medicine reviews, 7(2), 306–312. https://doi.org/10.1016/j.sxmr.2018.12.006

Scudellari M. (2015). Ageing research: Blood to blood. Nature, 517(7535), 426–429. https://doi.org/10.1038/517426a

Sha, SJ, Deutsch, GK, Tian, L., Richardson, K., Coburn, M., Gaudioso, JL, Marcal, T., Solomon, E., Boumis, A., Bet, A., Mennes, M ., van Oort, E., Beckmann, CF, Braithwaite, S. Jackson, S., Nikolich, K., Stephens, D., Kerchner, GA, & Wyss-Coray, T. (2019). Safety, Tolerability, and Feasibility of Young Plasma Infusion in the Plasma for Alzheimer Symptom Amelioration Study: A Randomized Clinical Trial. JAMA neurology, 76(1), 35–40. https://doi.org/10.1001/jamaneurol.2018.3288

Sharma, VK, Bhari, N., Patra, S., & Parihar, AS (2019). Platelet-Rich Plasma Therapy for Androgenetic Alopecia. Indian journal of dermatology, 64(5), 417-419. https://doi .org/10.4103/ijd.IJD_363_17

Smith, S. (2016) 10 Common Eldly Health Issues, Vital Record. Texas A&M Publication. https://vitalrecord.tamhsc.edu/10-common-elderly-health-issues/

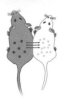

Stevens, J., & Khetarpal, S. (2018). Platelet-rich plasma for androgenetic alopecia: A review of the literature and proposed treatment protocol. International journal of women's dermatology, 5(1), 46–51. https:/ /doi.org/10.1016/j.ijwd.2018.08.004

Stowe, RP, Peek, MK, Cutchin, MP, & Goodwin, JS (2010). Plasma cytokine levels in a population-based study: relation to age and ethnicity. The journals of gerontology. Series A, Biological sciences and medical sciences, 65(4), 429-433. https://doi.org/10.1093/gerona/glp198.

Sun, Y., Shi, H., Yin, S., Ji, C., Zhang, X., Zhang, B., Wu, P., Shi, Y., Mao, F., Yan, Y., Xu, W., & Qian, H. (2018). Human Mesenchymal Stem Cell Derived Exosomes Alleviate Type 2 Diabetes Mellitus by Reversing Peripheral Insulin Resistance and Relieving β-Cell Destruction. ACS nano, 12(8), 7613–7628. https ://doi.org/10.1021/acsnano.7b07643

Taubes G. (2009). Insulin resistance. Prosperity's plague. Science (New York, NY), 325(5938), 256–260. https://doi.org/10.1126/science.325_256

Tavakol, S., Ashrafizadeh, M., Deng, S., Azarian, M., Abdoli, A., Motavaf, M., Poormoghadam, D., Khanbabaei, H., Afshar, EG, Mandegary, A., Pardakhty , A., Yap, CT, Mohammadinejad, R.,

& Kumar, AP (2019). Autophagy Modulators: Mechanistic Aspects and Drug Delivery Systems. Biomolecules, 9(10), 530. https://doi.org/10.3390/ biom9100530

Tompkins, BA, DiFede, DL, Khan, A., Landin, AM, Schulman, IH, Pujol, MV, Heldman, AW, Miki, R., Goldschmidt-Clermont, PJ, Goldstein, BJ, Mushtaq, M., Levis -Dusseau, S., Byrnes, JJ, Lowery, M., Natsumeda, M., Delgado, C., Saltzman, R., Vidro-Casiano, M., Da Fonseca, M., Golpanian, S., Hare, JM (2017). Allogeneic Mesenchymal Stem Cells Ameliorate Aging Frailty: A Phase II Randomized, Double-Blind, Placebo-Controlled Clinical Trial. The journals of gerontology. Series A, Biological sciences and medical sciences, 72(11), 1513–1522 . https://doi.org/10.1093/gerona/glx137

Tsoucalas, G. (2018) Dr Paul Niehans (1882-1971): Cell Therapy, the Secret of Life or a Life-Risking Trend? Archives of the Balkan Medical Union Vol. 53, Supplement 1

Tyagil, BPS, & Rout, M., (2019), Platelet Rich Plasma (PRP): A Revolutionary Treatment of Sensorineural Hearing Loss, Acta Scientific Otolaryngology 1.4: 02-05.

Ullah, M., Ng, NN, Concepcion, W., & Thakor, AS (2020). Emerging Role of Stem Cell-Derived Extracellular microRNAs in Age-Associated Human Diseases and in Different Therapies of

Longevity. Ageing Research Reviews, 57, 100979. https://doi.org/10.1016/j.arr.2019.100979

Van Velthoven, C. & Rando, TA (2019). Stem Cell Quiescence: Dynamism, Restraint, and Cellular Idling. Cell stem cell, 24(2), 213–225. https://doi.org/10.1016/j .stem. 2019.01.001

Vrselja, Z., Daniele, SG, Silbereis, J., Talpo, F., Morozov, YM, Sousa, A., Tanaka, BS, Skarica, M., Pletikos, M., Kaur, N., Zhuang, ZW , Liu, Z., Alkawadri, R., Sinusas, AJ, Latham, SR, Waxman, SG, & Sestan, N. (2019). Restoration of brain circulation and cellular functions hours post-mortem. Nature, 568(7752) , 336–343. https://doi.org/10.1038/s41586-019-1099-1

Weyand, CM, Goronzy, JJ (2016). Aging of the Immune System. Mechanisms and Therapeutic Targets. Annals of the American Thoracic Society, 13 Suppl 5 (Suppl 5), S422--S428. https://doi.org/10.1513 /AnnalsATS.201602-095AW

Whitmen, H. (2017) Erectile dysfunction: Stem cell therapy restores sexual function in phase I trial. https://www.medicalnewstoday.com/articles/316555

Wuxi Apptec (2018) Rejuvenation: The Role of Plasma Proteins in Counterbalancing Aging. https://wxpress.wuxiapptec.com/rejuvenation-role-plasma-proteins-counterbalancing-aging/

Xu, LL, Li, G. (2014) Circulating mesenchymal stem cells and their clinical implications, Journal of Orthopaedic Translation 2, 1e7

Zang, L., Hao, H., Liu, J., Li, Y., Han, W., & Mu, Y. (2017). Mesenchymal stem cell therapy in type 2 diabetes mellitus. Diabetology & metabolic syndrome, 9 , 36. https://doi.org/10.1186/s13098-017-0233-1

Zuk PA, Zhu M, Ashjian P, De Ugarte DA, Huang JI, Mizuno H, Alfonso ZC, Fraser JK, Benhaim P, Hedrick MH. (2002) Human adipose tissue is a source of multipotent stem cells. Mol Biol Cell. Dec ;13(12):4279-95. doi: 10.1091/mbc.e02-02-0105. PMID: 12475952; PMCID: PMC138633.